Ready, Set, GO!

SYNERGY FITNESS

for Time-Crunched Adults

Phil Campbell, M.S., M.A., ACSM-CPT, FACHE

Second Edition
Ninth Printing 2014

Pristine Publishers Inc. USA

Published by: Pristine Publishers Inc. USA
www.pristinepublishers.com
www.readysetgofitness.com
ISBN:10 0-9716633-8-6
ISBN:13 978-0-9716633-8-1
This book is the second edition, ninth printing of *Ready, Set, GO!*
Synergy Fitness for Time-Crunched Adults, printed in 2014.

This book is designed to provide information in regard to the subject matter covered for healthy adults. It is sold with the understanding that the publisher, author and advisors are not rendering medical advice or other professional services. It is highly recommended that an examination by a physician be performed BEFORE attempting to begin any fitness training programs outlined in this book.

The purpose of this book is to educate, expand thinking about fitness as an informational source for readers, and it is not medical advice, nor has it been evaluated by the FDA. The publisher, author, and advisors shall have neither liability nor responsibility to any person or entity with respect to any loss or damage caused or alleged to be caused directly or indirectly by the information and programs contained in this book. If you do not agree with the above, you may return to the publisher for a full refund.

SECOND EDITION, NINTH PRINTING, 2014
Printed in USA
Designed by Bruce Gore, Gore Studios, Nashville

Library of Congress Card Number 2001135854
Cataloging-in-Publication
    Campbell, Phil
    Ready, Set, GO!: Synergy Fitness for Time-Crunched Adults :
    a comprehensive fitness training guide for adults of all ages
    / Phil Campbell. -- 2nd ed.
    p. cm.
    Includes bibliographical references and index.
        ISBN 0-9716633-8-6

1. Physical fitness. 2. Exercise. 3. Health.
4. Aging--Prevention. I. Title.

RA781.C36 2002   613.7
                        QBI02-953

Contents

Part 3   *GO!*

Foreword

by Marilyn DeMartini

"Ready, set, go!" Remember the glee as you yelled those words, then tore down the street with wild abandon, breathless as you raced your buddies to the end of the block?

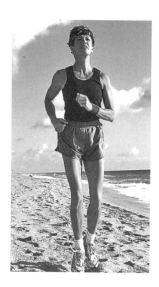

Ready, Set, GO! Synergy Fitness can rekindle those emotions for adults, recapturing the rush of pushing to the maximum, to achieve the optimum.

"How do you stay motivated to work out so hard and so often?" People often ask. "Fear," I reply.

Fear of 40, now of 50, the fat little Italian girl I imagine chasing me has been a constant and powerful motivator - especially with age. Why have I seemed to be working harder, not to make progress, but only to maintain?

Why does aging bring with it the albatross of lagging energy, sagging skin and body fat? Why have I refused to accept that fate? Because along with age, comes wisdom, and I have learned that staying fit fights aging.

Now, with Phil Campbell's help, I understand how to work smarter, not just harder - how to use and understand science to build a tactical defense in my war against aging.

Marilyn DeMartini has worked as a sports and fitness journalist covering sports apparel, gear and health trends for over a decade. She has recently written major articles about anti-aging, functional training and sports medicine for many national publications.

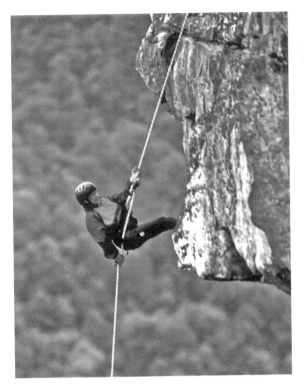

Technology's response to the fight to stay young has not just been in digital treadmills and talking heart monitors. Technology brings real science and research that help us better understand how our bodies   work - and don't.

Campbell brings this scientific proof to readers in a clear and concise way, explaining clinical studies on nutrition, energy production and exercise - showing how *Ready, Set, GO! Fitness* makes sense, *why* it works.

Optimal fitness and the coincidental path to anti-aging are not about languishing on a treadmill for hours or struggling with overly heavy barbells. Ready, Set Go, Synergy Fitness is about getting the most out of your workout by putting the most into it - by leading the body to generate and release its own   anti-aging formula - human growth hormone.

As a journalist, fitness enthusiast and instructor, I have studied trends, research and ideology and reported on what to wear, take and do, to stay fit. The recent research and exposure of (HGH) human growth hormone's effect on performance has created a major breakthrough in health and anti-aging medicine.

While athletes, movie stars and those with clinical deficiency take injections to counteract age-related HGH decline, Campbell presents a plan to self-induce HGH release, resetting our biological clocks through high-intensity exercise, a "Sprint" 8 program.

To be healthy, it is not enough to be thin or not to be sick. Real health takes a commitment to *feel* your own body - listen to its messages - follow its instinct, and then, enjoy the uplift. The energy generated by pushing your body to its maximum lasts throughout the day and throughout a lifetime. Better than looking good <u>for</u> your age is *feeling* good - <u>at</u> your age.

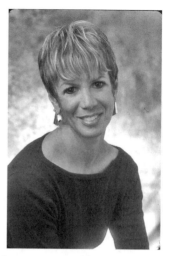

When at the top of your physical game, you'll be at the top of your mental game - tying together the elements of feeling and staying young. Feeling fatigued, unattractive, sleep-deprived and achy, the overweight and under-exercised majority may tell us that it is the reality of aging - just middle age catching up with us.

On the contrary, some of us have decided to run from old age - literally. And run at a full sprint!

Not into running? Then walk fast, bike, skate - even dance - as long as you do it with passion and intensity. Mix that emotion with inexpensive, easy-to-obtain supplements and go at your chosen aerobic activity until you're breathless - anaerobic.

The Sprint 8 program will take you to new heights in your fitness level and in your attitude. Science and experience show how to arm our bodies for the war against aging. Campbell shows how to make it simple and even fun.

If you are content to accept an expanding waistline, a waning energy level, decreased sex drive or general feeling of malaise, this book is not for you. But, if you want to look and feel great at any age, follow the *Ready, Set, Go! Fitness* plan. This simple book asks only for you to give it a try. Kick your body into full gear and tap your own Fountain of Youth. It's not in a bottle. It's in your veins.

About the Author

If you've seen a fitness magazine lately like *Oprah's O Magazine, Outside Magazine, Physical Magazine, OnFitness, Ms. Fitness, Muscle Mag*, or Brian Mackenzie's *Successful Coaching*, you may have seen an article or a quote by masters athlete and author Phil Campbell, MS., M.A, Certified American College of Sports Medicine.

You may have seen him on the cover of *Personal Fitness Professional*, or heard him speak during the *Health & Fitness Expo* in Denver or during Greta Blackburn's *Malibu Fit Camp*.

You may own a piece of award-winning Vision Fitness cardio equipment featuring his *Sprint 8* program. Or you may know an athlete who has traveled

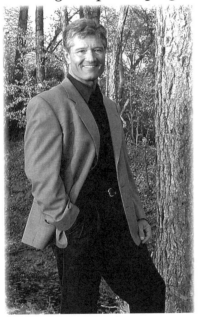

internationally to him for advanced speed technique training. But until you've read his book, you may have missed the most meaningful fitness improvement experience of your life. His book is that good!

Phil Campbell holds two advanced degrees, and he is board certified by ACHE. He applies his advanced degree training in Health Services and his years of experience in the development of *Ready, Set, Go! Synergy Fitness.*

Not only does he bring 38 years of experience training individuals and athletes to this project, he also brings 20 years experience in hospital administration where it was his responsibility to take the medical disciplines of surgery, pathology, radiology, pediatrics, physical rehabilitation, physical therapy, pharmacology, and other health disciplines and operationalize diverse medical services into a comprehensive healthcare delivery system that improved the lives of others. And he has taken that same approach in the presentation of information to his readers.

Phil Campbell uses 300 photo-illustrations and cites over 200 mainstream research studies in the biomedical disciplines of endocrinology, exercise science, medicine, and fitness training for specific age groups to present a research-supported system that will help improve the lives of others.

Phil Campbell has a gift for taking complex medical subjects and making them understandable and practical. He shows readers step-by-step how to improve fitness, increase energy, lose, cut, and tone in the most efficient way possible.

Phil Campbell wrote his first fitness training manual over 30 years ago. While in college, he managed health clubs and performed personal training ... 20 years before it was called personal training.

His inspiration to help improve the health status of large populations was sparked by his Health Services advanced degree advisor, Dr. Ed Cavanaugh, a former division administrator with the Centers for Disease Control in Atlanta. Mainstream biomedical research is the basis for all of Phil Campbell's writing, and over 200 research studies are cited in his book.

As a masters athlete, Phil Campbell holds several USA Track and Field Masters titles including first place in the 100-meter sprint, Southeastern US Championships for his age group in 2000. In 2003, he won the 200-meter sprint and the discus throw, placed second in the 100 meters, and he set the meet record in the javelin during the USA Masters Track & Field Tennessee Championships.

Nationally, he has placed third in USA Track and Field Masters Nationals in his age group in the javelin, and fifth in discus. In his late 40s, he won a 40-yard dash open competition in 4.69 seconds. He teaches athletes how to improve speed, agility and quickness during his Speed Camps - www.40speed.com. He holds a black belt in Isshinryu Karate and has competed and won first place in martial arts and weightlifting competitions.

Thousands of people across the US have been inspired by Phil Campbell's motivational presentation "Fitness for a Lifetime."

If you'll let him, Phil Campbell will show you how to have the most successful and lasting fitness improvement experience of your life.

PRISTINE PUBLISHERS INC. USA

What Others are Saying About this Book...

I predict Campbell's book will become the next fitness best-seller.
- Joanna Daneman, Amazon Top 10 Reviewer

I absolutely guarantee you will NOT be able to put this book down.
-Thomas Woodrow, What You Need to Know About Running

5 Stars. Superbly presented.
Profusely illustrated.
Practical and Effective.
Highly Recommended!
- Midwest Book Reviews

Ready, Set, Go! Synergy Fitness explains why so many people start exercising, don't see results and give up. The program is easy to understand, has transformed people of all fitness levels and ages, and is supported by more scientific research than I've seen in any other consumer fitness book. **- Vera Tweed, health and fitness writer**

Ready, Set, GO! Synergy Fitness is a real breakthrough in the health industry. His recommendations are sound and exercise routines are extremely effective. I highly recommend his book.
-Chad Tackett, CPT Fitness Expert
- Global Health and Fitness http://www.global-fitness.com

I now understand why even the best diet and regular weight lifting weren't working. With a few tweaks to my workout program (and no more time involvement), I have twice the energy and feel more toned than I've felt in a long time. **- Nan Allison, MS, RD, License Nutritionist Author of *Full and Fulfilled***

I could be a spokesperson for you! This has literally changed my entire life! I have lost 130 pounds so far. With what I've learned from your book, I have seen more results in one week than in 2 years doing "conventional" exercise!!! ! Thank you!!!
- **Debbie Gross, Wilmington, Delaware**

This book is brilliant!
- **Mike Gotfredson**
President, Road
Runner Sports

Phil Campbell has discovered the secret to maximizing exercise potential. His book does it all. It provides the most comprehensive exercise plans I have seen to date. And I have tried virtually every type of program that has come out in the past 30 years. It seemed as I got older, positive results were impossible to achieve, impossible that is, until I began following the step-by-step Ready, Set, Go! Fitness program. This plan can turn back the clock for anyone. It has changed my life both physically and mentally! - **Detective Captain Mickey Miller**

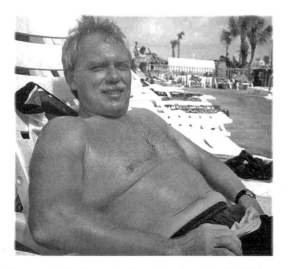 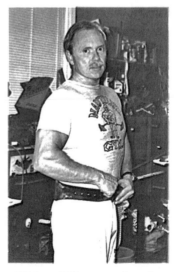

One week before starting *Ready, Set, Go! Fitness*   Mickey Miller - 90 days later

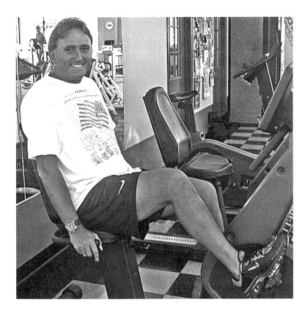

I'm glad I bought this book. Even with bad knees I found that I can still do the Sprint 8 Workout on the bike at the gym. In a few short weeks, I lost 10 pounds. And I didn't have to diet.
- Dr. Steve Kail

This is the fitness program I do personally, and I highly recommend it. **- Dr. Keith Atkins**

At my age of 55, I have felt frustrated by a lowered metabolism and energy level. The growth hormone release was new information for me. Acquiring an understanding of the HGH release has made a significant difference in my weight loss success. Not only do I feel healthier, but I have lost those 20 pounds in just 10 weeks!
- Pauline Blanchard, Salt Lake City, Utah

Ready, Set, Go! Fitness works! Phil Campbell has taken the lead in training techniques, general fitness and nutrition.
- Dr. L. Schrader, Orthopedic Surgeon

Campbell's qualifications make his routine an easy sell. The author is a twenty-year veteran in the healthcare field, including a stint as a division president in charge of eight hospitals. He is also an accom-

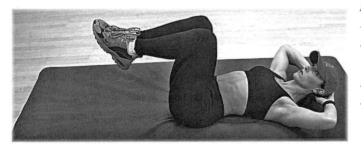

plished athlete who holds several USA Track and Field Masters titles as well as a black belt in Is-shinryu Karate.
- Forward Reviews

The next fitness revolution is here and it's called Ready, Set, Go! Fitness. I was finishing my masters in Exercise Science when Aerobics fired the shot that started the world running and ushered in the "Cardio" revolution. Ready, Set, Go! Fitness is destined to change fitness training as we know it today.
- **Alvin Hoover, FACHE**
  Hospital Administrator
  South Carolina

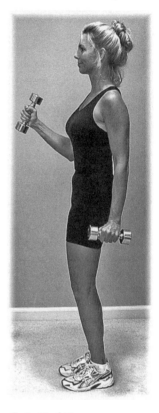

This is an excellent fitness workbook...Along with photos of people performing the actual exercise, there are explicit descriptions of how the exercise should be done correctly and why. I've already used this book to add to my usual exercise routine. I think it's improved my overall performance dramatically! I recommend this book for everyone young and old!
- **Lisa, Managing Editor**
  THE BOOK REVIEW CAFE

Phil Campbell, M.S., M.A., in his excellent book, Ready, Set, Go! Synergy Fitness, outlines the detailed exercise (weight training, sprinting, plyometrics, stretching, drills, including hundreds of photos), and supplements to produce growth hormone by natural means and thus improve athletic performance and increase longevity. Phil Campbell, a very fit muscular 52 year old athlete is the living example of his book. His methods are backed up by frequent reference to many scientific studies in this area. An ideal easy-to-apply book for triathletes, swimmers, cyclists, runners, and fitness advocates."
- **Earl Fee, Author of**
  The Complete Guide to Running

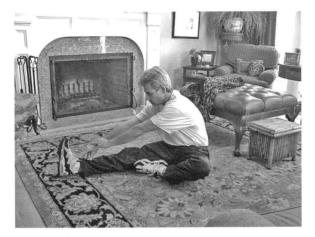

Dr. Williams performing the 10-Minute Stretching Routine

As a physician, I recognize and encourage patients in the importance of exercise and nutrition and the benefits obtained from a sustained program. But like most, I struggle with the ability to maintain an exercise program. For two decades I have tried multiple programs but have been frustrated by the time commitment, expense, isolated results, and lack of desired results for maintaining overall physical health.

After reading this book, I started the Ready, Set, Go! Fitness program. I was amazed at the results I achieved in body flexibility, strength, endurance, and improvement in overall sense of well being that results from a regular exercise program. Most of all I was able to accomplish this with a reasonable time investment, because I was able to do the program on my time at home.

This plan is practical, scientifically based, and meets my goals for good health now and into the future.

- Dr. Keith Williams, Ob-Gyn

BOOXS Review of Good Books

Lean and mean workbook outlining Campbell's Synergy Fitness plan for time-crunched adults, a fluffless, step-by-step guide that promises four main how-to's: Increasing the body's anti-aging growth hormone naturally; looking years younger while achieving optimum health and fitness, developing a sprinter's physique at any age; and rediscovering the energy of youth.

A well-illustrated and explained in-your-face rant that pushes the aerobics crowd to an all new level. **- Geoff Rotunno, Managing Editor**

I have been athletic all my life, but with the addition of the Sprint 8 and E-Lifts, I am no doubt in the best shape of my life at age 39.
The addition of the Ready, Set, Go! Fitness E-Lifting techniques to my workout enabled me to increase my bench by 20 percent in just 6 weeks. I receive compliments daily on my new found physique.
Bring on Age 40!

- Jeff Mitchell, President
  Benefit Consulting Services

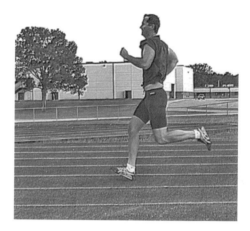

Heartland Reviews

Ready, Set, Go! Synergy Fitness is the fitness book for us middle-aged baby boomers. It focuses on the natural re-energizing of our bodies growth hormone production, which is critical for anti-aging.
It is sensibly written and has an immense amount of research data to back up everything it advises. Where this book is different from many is in its focus on the intensity of exercise which is required to see results and in the importance of planning and timing. This guide takes a whole-body and a varied type-exercise approach to fitness.
The author is a highly qualified expert who gives out trustworthy, knowledgeable guidance.
This is like having your own personal trainer.

  - Bob Spear, Publisher Heartland Reviews

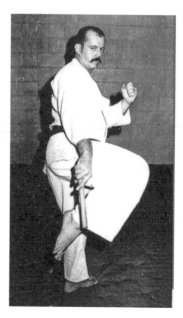

Bob Spear (right, 1975 photo) is a nationally recognized self-defense expert. He is a 7th degree black belt in Hapkido,

What Triathletes are Saying

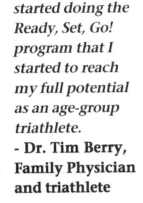

I have read every book on training for triathlons, but it was not until I started doing the Ready, Set, Go! program that I started to reach my full potential as an age-group triathlete.
- Dr. Tim Berry, Family Physician and triathlete

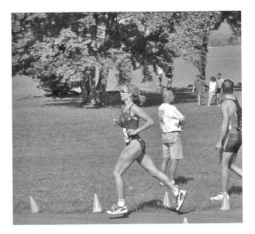

Dr. Debra Berry, Pediatrician completing a triathlon

As a former elite athlete who still wants to compete on a high level in master's cycling events, I have incorporated the Sprint 8 Workout as a key component of my weekly training program. The Sprint 8 Workout definitely offers significant positive fitness returns in the sport of cycling which requires the use of all three muscle types.
- Tom Gee, Age 50, triathlete and national cycling title holder

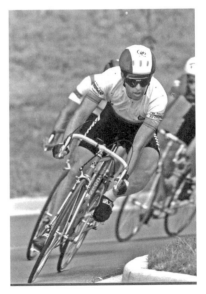

Tom Gee qualified for two Olympic trials. He is a five time medalist in the US Cycling National Masters Championships; four time finisher of Paris-Brest-Paris; and a veteran of two world championships, and 11 European road races

After being a competitive runner for over 36 years, I thought that there was little more that I could learn. I was totally wrong! Ready, Set, Go! Synergy Fitness has revolutionized my training and I can't thank Phil enough.

I have lost body fat, gained energy and strength and I am running better than I have in years. Phil's book shows you how to incorporate his training methods into your bicycling, swimming, running or other cardiovascular workout as well as maximize the benefit that you get from your strength workout.

You owe it to yourself to order this book and start achieving all of the goals that you have always wanted to, but never been able to achieve.
- Rich Drafter, Howtobefit.com

I want to take the time to tell you how much I enjoyed the book. You were able to take complicated subject matter and reduce it into layman's terms. I am 38 years old and have been exercising for two years on a regular basis. I couldn't agree with you more. I used to worry that maybe my running was impeding muscle growth. However, reading your book has convinced me about the benefits of anaerobic exercise. Thanks.
- Joseph Donofrio, New Jersey

Book Review
Ready, Set, GO! Synergy Fitness
by Dwayne Hines, II, CPT, national fitness writer

This book is a total departure from the traditional approach to fat loss!

It takes an effective stab at the prevailing wisdom in the fitness world. Ready Set Go Fitness is a revolutionary concept for fat loss and lean muscularity. Campbell focuses on the key area of HGH growth hormone release through two familiar channels—diet and exercise, but via unconventional means.

This is a radical new approach to shaping the ultimate physique. It contains the program for drastically changing your body for the better. The book is full of various weight training exercises,

plyometrics, sprinting and stretching exercises to provide the body with a total package.

*For those who want to ramp up their training and take it to the next
level, Ready, Set, Go! Synergy Fitness is a proven way to do it.*
- **Cary Nosler, Host, Wide World of Health KSTE Talk Radio,**

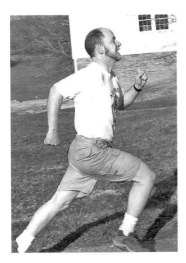

*Phil Campbell's book, Ready, Set, Go!
Synergy Fitness is a concise, well
researched, practical program for
people of all ages.
After following the level 2 program for
8 weeks, my total cholesterol dropped
from 221 to 157. Because of its
principle-based teaching and structured
guidelines, I highly recommend this
book to my patients, and they receive
reproducible results.*
- **Dr. Chet Gentry, Family Physician**

*I just wanted to tell you how much I am enjoying your book and your
philosophy about exercise. I am sharing it with co-workers and clients.
It makes so much sense and I can see using it to supplement and/or
replace our current approach to working with many...if not all....clients.*
- **Deborah Tregea M.Ed, Senior Exercise Physiologist University
Fitness Center, Penn State Hershey Medical Center**

*After not quite 3 months on your program, I've now burned about
19 pounds of fat, added about 4 pounds of muscle, and cut body fat by
almost 6 percent. I'm tremendously grateful for your insights and am
turning friends on to your book and ideas at every opportunity. I had a
complete physical this morning and even my doctor was impressed. My
cholesterol dropped 70 points (to 207 since my last test 2 years ago!!)
I am stronger than I've ever been in my life and fitter than I've been
in at least a decade.*
- **Terry Bazyluk, Writer/Lawyer, Maryland**

What Others are Saying About this Book ... Internationally

Ready Set Go, Synergy Fitness, uses revolutionary research and a sound scientific approach, to offer a practical and effective way to help middle age adults, and adults of all ages get fit and stay young.
- **Stefan Angheli, CSCS, Editor, HealthFitness.com, Australia**

The workout to accelerate GH release works. I am 69 years old. After a few months of practicing I feel the tightness of muscles built in my buttocks and thighs that gives me a feeling of youth I never experienced even when I was young. - **Chi On Kwan, Hong Kong**

I love this book - it's brilliant - very readable - and it all makes sense!
- **Dickon Weir-Hughes, Deputy CEO & Chief Nurse Royal Marsden Hospital, London, United Kingdom**

I'm really glad that I discovered Ready, Set, GO! Fitness. I'm 38, have never had much exercise, and yet I'm running. Your book inspired me. My weight has dropped and seems to have leveled out at 9 stone (122 pounds). This program is fabulous. The most noticeable difference is that I look and feel healthier and my muscles are beginning to tone.
- **Sally Somerville, Channel Islands, United Kingdom**

Ready, Set, GO! Synergy Fitness is a practical, science-based fitness plan anyone can use to lose weight, delay the middle-age "somatopause," and boost their anti-aging hormones naturally.
Phil Campbell's book is an easy-to-use, step-by-step plan for anyone who wants to turn back the clock and look their very best - no matter what their age. I highly recommend it!
- **Christian Finn, M.Sc., Northampton, United Kingdom**

Fitness America Pageant Winner & Ms. Natural Olympia Dena Anne Weiner

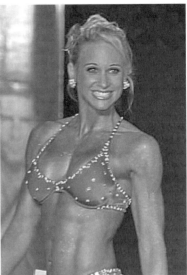

Dena Anne Weiner, 43, Ms. Natural Olympia Fitness, and national fitness champion uses the Ready, Set, Go! Fitness anaerobic sprint workouts during her training and competition preparation

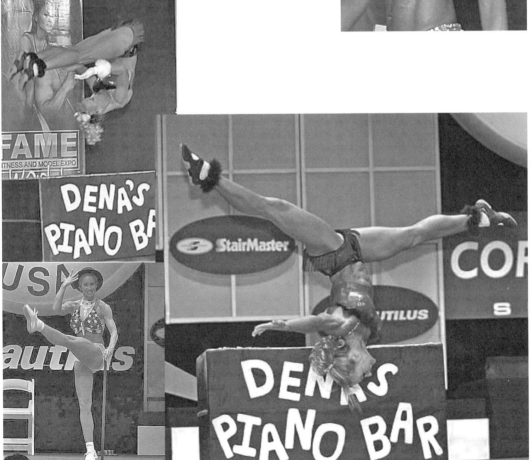

Book Review
by Anthony Yniguez "Mr. Why"
Catholic School principal in Azusa, CA

This is an excellent fitness book. It is both well researched and well written. What makes this book so good is the fact that if you follow the program the author is outlining, then you will cover every aspect of fitness that is important, the author does not leave anything out. From weigthlifting, to cardio, to stretching, to anaerobic interval style training, everything is present in this program. I have read many other books that make an argument that weightlifting is essential, but leave out how to integrate cardio work. Some books emphasize cardio, but leave out the short "sprint" style interval training that is so important to overall fitness. This plan covers everything!

I read the book twice and love the illustrations, the motivation, and the research that you share. I read lots of books on exercise, nutrition, and diabetes in particular. Your book is at the top of my motivational reading! - **Darrell Denman, WI**

Phil Campbell's book is one of the most informative, well researched, and beneficial books I've read. - **Rory Karpf, producer with NFL Films**

Phil Campbell is not trying to sell you anything except a longer, healthier life. A terrific concept, easy read, and a welcomed addition to a health and fitness library filled with more style than substance. This is the real deal.
- **Keith Murphy, NBC Sports Director, Des Moines**

"Awesome book! Thank you so much for putting your discovery and research together in a clear, concise and easy to follow book." - **Bruce Lippiatt**

I have just finished reading Ready, Set, GO, Synergy Fitness and wish to complement you on authoring such a superb book. No fluff, no outrageous claims, just solid material from cover to cover. The material on HGH is very exciting, to say the least." - **Renzo Caredda**

Acknowledgments

It is an honor to recognize, and publicly thank key individuals who contributed to the creation, development and production of the second edition of this book.

I want to thank my children Holly, Christine and John for serving as *Ready, Set, Go! Fitness* demonstrators and reminding me of the really important things in life. From the initial encouragement to write the book, to taking photo-illustrations, to proofreading text, I want to thank my wife, Kathy, for her contributions and commitment to this project. And thanks to my Mom, Bertha McClenny, for her unconditional love and support.

I am indebted to many for their contributions: Bruce Gore for book cover and interior design, editors Dr. Lorraine Singer, Jean Norville, Pat Thomson, Maria Hasz, and Paula Hoover played major roles in this book.

Authors Dr. Randall Bush, Nan Allison and Pat Winston are to be recognized for their coaching along with personal trainers Bambi LaFont, Melanie Buchholz, and others who took part in demonstrating *Ready, Set, Go! Fitness* techniques. Special thanks to the University School of Jackson and to my training partners Nate Robertson, Terry Bumpus, and the others who assisted with the production of this book.

My Health Services masters degree advisor, Dr. Ed Cavanaugh, a former division administrator with the Centers for Disease Control in Atlanta needs to be recognized for his inspiration and instruction concerning the way to approach improving health status of large populations - go to the source of the problem to find the solution.

Lastly, this book is dedicated to biomedical researchers. Frequently, researchers are listed in bibliographies tucked in the back of books. Writers cite study findings in a few brief moments without fully appreciating the years of hard work it took to produce the study results.

Seldom do researchers receive the recognition they deserve for the significant impact they have on the lives of others. For this reason, research boxes are added inside the book beside the topic discussed so readers can see the study and the lead researcher performing the study.

~ Phil Campbell

Welcome to
Ready, Set, GO! Fitness

This book is about "exercise-induced growth hormone," what it is; what it does; and most importantly, how you can produce more of the most powerful fat-burning, muscle-toning, fitness-improving substance known in science.

It's estimated that 500,000 adults are injecting growth hormone for its amazing benefits. Growth hormone has been banned from athletes because it can significantly enhance performance. For middle-age and older adults, growth hormone is described as the fitness hormone and the fountain of youth. Descriptions of this substance include every positive adjective imaginable to picture unlimited high-energy youthfulness.

On average, injecting growth hormone can pull off 28 pounds of body fat from a 200-pound adult. And it can add 8 percent lean mass. We're talking about a powerful substance.

This book is not about getting the benefits of growth hormone from injections. The purpose of this book is to show you how to get the best form of growth hormone - not from injecting it - but from producing it naturally within your own body. New research shows that certain forms of exercise, adequate "deep sleep," and some inexpensive nutritional supplements, like 2-grams of L-glutamine, can significantly increase your body's release of this hormone.

Along with discovering how you can help your body produce more of this hormone, you'll learn how to avoid some things that can hinder, and even stop, its production.

You'll also discover how to maximize exercise-induced growth hormone once it's released so that you can receive the benefits of growth hormone produced by your own body.

"The exercise-induced secretion of GH (growth hormone) plays a significant role in the regulation of fatty acid metabolism." (Acute exposure to GH during exercise stimulates the turnover of free fatty acids in GH - deficient men, 2004, J Appl Physiol, Kanaley).

"Exercise is a potent, dose-dependent stimulus of growth hormone (GH) secretion."

(Acute Exercise has no Effect on Ghrelin Plasma Concentrations, J Horm Metab Res, 2004, Schmit).

Exercise-induced growth hormone targets and burns body fat like a guided missile for two hours. And this book will provide you with fitness improvement strategies that will help you receive all the fat burning, muscle toning, and building benefits available from this incredible substance.

Multi-Tasking Saves Time

Ready, Set, GO! Synergy Fitness will not only show you how to increase exercise-induced growth hormone, it will also show you how to combine several forms of exercises to save time.

This is called "multi-tasking" exercises. It's a time-saver for "time-crunched adults." Best of all, multi-tasking gets great results.

Five Fitness Levels

There are five different fitness plans in this book. They are matched with five different fitness levels that are based on age, current fitness status, and training experience.

"The beneficial effects of exercise can mimic and are not additive to the effects of GH treatment alone."

(Exercise training benefits growth hormone (GH)-deficient adults in absence or presence of GH treatment, 2003, J Clin Endocrinol Metab, Thomas SG).

You'll need to place yourself into one of the five Fitness Level categories before you begin. As you read, be thinking about the category that would be best for you. Having five Fitness Levels means that beginners, all the way to advanced athletes, will have a plan to meet their needs.

Fitness for a Lifetime

Ready, Set, Go! Fitness seeks to provide you with the most exciting and productive fitness improvement experience ever! The goal is for you to experience so many wonderful benefits that you'll continue after the initial eight-week commitment. And the great results will keep you motivated for a lifetime.

Sections in the Book

Ready, Set, Go! Synergy Fitness sticks to one philosophy of cutting through the fads and gimmicks and delivers real information that you can begin using immediately.

Ready, Set, Go! Synergy Fitness will bring you all the excitement and action of a race. Just before the race begins, you may hear the loud words: **Ready . . . Set**, and on **GO!**, the action explodes. This book follows that same course.

The first two sections of the book prepare you for the greatest fitness improvement experience of your life. The information in these sections will have you **READY** and **SET** to implement one of five levels of **Strategic Fitness Plans** in the **GO** section of this book.

"No Wasted Time, No Gimmicks and No Fluff!"

If you are a time-crunched adult as I am, you probably thumb through magazines and books to determine if the information is worth reading. Let me assure you that the time you spend with this book will yield significant health, fitness, appearance, and energy dividends. However, before the race begins, there are the *Ready* and *Set* phases that must be accomplished before the runner is allowed to race.

Let me encourage you not to jump to the *Go* phase without first going through the *Ready* and *Set* phases. You'll miss crucially important information if you do!

HELPFUL RESEARCH

As you go through this book, you will see shaded boxes like this in the margins. These boxes contain supporting bio-medical research information. Research Boxes allow you to see the reliability of the information and the date of the scientific research. Over 200 research studies are cited in this book.

The New England Journal of Medicine published a study showing human growth hormone replacement therapy increased muscle mass by 8.8 percent and decreased fat by 14.4 percent in older adults. (Rudman).

Why Are Famous Actors, Athletes, and Bodybuilders Taking Hormones?

Recent discoveries about hormones, particularly human growth hormone (HGH), are changing the way scientists think about fitness, health, athletic performance, aging, and even middle-aging. The benefits of the research discoveries apply to athletes of all ages, patients at anti-aging centers, and middle-aged adults trying to lose weight, get in shape, and restore the energy of their youth.

Children with severe growth problems have been treated with human growth hormone effectively for many years; it makes them grow taller and stronger. HGH will not, however, make adults grow taller.

Growth hormone injections can improve athletic performance so they have been banned for athletes. Injecting growth hormone can pull off 14 percent body fat, add 8 percent lean muscle mass, and do many other positive things to the body, so anti-aging centers promote HGH injections as the fountain of youth.

From *USA Today* to Oprah

"...exercise is a powerful stimulus to GH release." (Neuroendocrine control of GH release during acute aerobic exercise, 2003, J Endocrinol Invest, Weltman A).

The anti-aging benefits of HGH replacement therapy via injections have been touted, and rightfully so - the impact of increasing HGH is nothing less than miraculous!

Medical researchers attempting to delay the effects of aging have treated adults with the same HGH therapy used for treating growth problems in children. The results are phenomenal. Injecting human growth hormone into adults was found to reverse the effects of aging that were reported to be equivalent to 10 to 20 years of aging.

Today, some researchers are also debating the concept of using growth hormone therapy to delay what increasingly is being referred to as the "somatopause" (sa-mot-a-pause). This is the metabolic slow-down and weight-gain phase of middle-age that is sometimes called the "middle-age spread."

The rush of "baby-boomers" experiencing the somatopause - attempting to drink from the "fountain of youth" by receiving HGH injections - is, thus, an understandable phenomenon. But what if there is a way to get the benefits of HGH - without injections? Well, there is, and that's what this book intends to show you!

You will learn how you can increase HGH (your fitness hormone) naturally without the potentially risky side-effects of HGH injections!

The discovery that HGH can be increased naturally with specific types of exercise will revolutionize the health and fitness world during the next decade. You can get so much more than the calorie-burning benefits of exercise by performing the type of fitness training that increases your body's natural release of HGH. Synergy is possible when you exercise to release HGH.

There is no need for potentially harmful HGH injections for most adults. With the correct fitness plan, which is aimed at increasing HGH naturally in your body, you will be able to improve your fitness, health, appearance, and energy by leaps and bounds. You will be able to cut body fat and inches, lose weight, tone and build muscle, and feel great!

This book can be your guide to achieving new levels of health, fitness, and appearance. The first step is to commit to following one of the five Strategic Fitness Plans for an initial eight-week period.

"Exercise is a potent stimulus for the release human growth hormone (HGH)." (Growth hormone response to a repeated maximal cycle ergometer exercise at different pedaling rates." 2002, Stokes).

"Exercise has a profound effect on the release of human growth hormone." (Growth hormone and exercise, 1999, Jenkins).

The Fitness Evolution

In our fast-paced world, new information constantly impacts our lives daily. At breakneck speed, we see medicine, science, and technology moving to ever new and higher levels of understanding and insight.

Medical knowledge, believed to be advanced only a few years ago, can even generate malpractice claims today.

The first comprehensive book on medicine in sports, *Hygiene des Sports,* by Sigfried Weissbein, was published in 1910. It discussed the effects of exercise on the body, injuries, and age-specific recommendations. Not until 1979 were sports physiology and training methods - acceleration sprints, circuit training, and running intervals - applied to sports training.

Fitness training has been evolving for some time toward a comprehensive fitness model that uses strategies and planning principles. In fitness centers across the world, there are discussions of "cardio" after weight training. Marathoners now recognize the value in running intervals and weight training. Bodybuilders now see the importance of stretching between sets and using stepping machines for cardio. Why? Results, that's why! But could they do even better? I say, "yes!"

There is one key component missing in most fitness plans today. It is the need for anaerobic exercise. This is the quick-burst, short, get-you-out-of-breath type of exercise. Sprinting, high-intensity interval training, sprint swimming, sprint cycling, XC skiing, sprint skating, and even sprint power walking qualifies as anaerobic - if it gets you out-of-breath and fatigues you quickly.

Anaerobic exercise should be a major focus in your fitness plan because it's absolutely essential for releasing exercise-induced growth hormone in your body.

If you are not a runner, don't be frightened by words like "sprints" and "running." There are many other methods (and one just right for you) of performing anaerobic exercise.

"CONCLUSIONS: Total physical activity and vigorous activities showed the strongest reductions in CHD (coronary heart disease) *risk. Moderate and light activities, which may be less precisely measured, showed nonsignificant inverse associations."* (Physical activity and coronary heart disease in men: The Harvard Alumni Health Study. Circulation. 2000 Aug 29, Sesso HD).

You can change your appearance with anaerobic exercise. I want you to take a common-sense test. The next time track and field, Olympic swimming, or speed-skating is on TV, look at the sprinting athletes. Notice their physiques.

Why are sprinters (in every sport) lean, muscular, and so healthy in appearance? Research is now confirming what sprinters have always known about anaerobic exercise! Anaerobic exercise pulls off body fat, puts on muscle, and makes you feel great (after the workout, of course).

New research discoveries explain why sprinters look the way they do. Research clearly shows that the short-burst types of anaerobic exercise that sprinters perform will make the body release significant amounts of growth hormone. And lower intensities of exercise will not. It's that simple!

For years, the gold standard for exercise has been *30 minutes of activity a day*. And walking for 30 minutes a day was said to be adequate enough to delay heart disease and premature death. Researchers now disagree.

A new study involving 2,000 men over 10 years destroys the low-intensity, walking standard. Researchers show that low-intensity does nothing to prevent death from heart disease.

Nearly 2,000 men, ages 45 to 59, were tracked for 10 years. Initially, none of the men had any evidence of heart disease. Exercise was performed and measured by three levels of intensity: low, moderate, and high. Low-intensity included walking & bowling. Golf & dancing qualified as moderate-intensity. And running & swimming were ranked as high-intensity.

Of the 252 deaths that occurred during the 10-year study, 75% were linked to heart disease and stroke. And cancer accounted for 25%. Conclusion: Walking 30 minutes five times a week is not enough to prevent early death from heart disease. Moderate-intensity also failed to reduce premature deaths. Only the highest levels of exercise intensity lowered death rates.

"vigorous activities but not nonvigorous activities were associated with longevity." (Exercise intensity and longevity in men. The Harvard Alumni Health Study. JAMA. 1995 Apr 19, Lee IM).

"exercise classified as heavy or vigorous was independently associated with reduced risk of premature death from CVD (cardiovascular disease)." (What level of physical activity protects against premature cardiovascular death? The Caerphilly study. Heart. 2003 May, Yu S).

Approximately 250,000 Americans die prematurely due to physical inactivity. (Waging war on modern chronic diseases: primary prevention through exercise biology, 2000, Booth).

Degrees of Health and Fitness

The worldwide fitness movements of weight training in the 1960s and distance running in the 1980s were effective for compulsive individuals who made time for an hour or two of training every day. However, many Americans were left behind during these fitness revolutions.

As a result, obesity in the United States is now widespread and is increasing at an alarming rate. According to a report by the Centers for Disease Control (CDC) concerning health status in America, not one state had an obesity rate above 15 percent in 1987.

Four years later (as channel surfing was becoming a national pastime), six states, in less than 10 years, had reached this level.

By 2001, the national obesity rate had reached 22 percent. What does this mean? Nearly one in four Americans is obese, and 61 percent of adults are overweight. Now, the second most common cause of *actual death* is "poor diet and lack of exercise."

In a study of elderly subjects (average age 79), researchers conclude that enriched food has no effect on improving the immune system. However, "exercise may prevent or slow the age-related decline in immune response." (Immunity in frail elderly: a randomized controlled trial of exercise and enriched foods, 2000, Paw).

The situation has become so critical that the U.S. Surgeon General stated, "Overweight and obesity may soon cause as much preventable disease and death as cigarette smoking."

There are 300,000 deaths a year associated with overweight and obesity compared to 400,000 deaths related to tobacco. The estimated cost of these public health menaces combined runs $117 billion per year (*Overweight and Obesity Threaten U.S. Health Gains*, December 12, 2001, HHS), and the costs show no sign of slowing.

Being overweight causes cancer reports medical researchers. Obesity and the medical condition of being "overweight" now account for 14 to 20% of deaths by cancer (*Overweight, obesity, and mortality from cancer in a prospectively studied cohort of US adults*, 2003, Calle).

This wasn't a small, out-of-context study conducted over a few months. Over 900,000 adults were studied for 16 years. Researchers estimated that more than 90,000 cancer deaths each year could be avoided if every American maintained a healthy weight. The researchers concluded:

> *We estimate that current patterns of overweight and obesity in the U.S. could account for 14 percent of all deaths from cancer in men and 20 percent of those in women.* (2003, Calle).

This study also shows that the risk of dying from cancer is 52% higher for overweight men than for men of normal weight. It is 62% higher for women. All the more reason to start and maintain a lifestyle that makes fitness training a priority.

"The importance of GH in most physiological systems suggests that GH deficiency at any age would be associated with significant morbidity." (Growth hormone therapy and Quality of Life: possibilities, pitfalls and mechanisms, J Endocrinol, 2003 Dec, Hull KL).

Actual Causes of Death

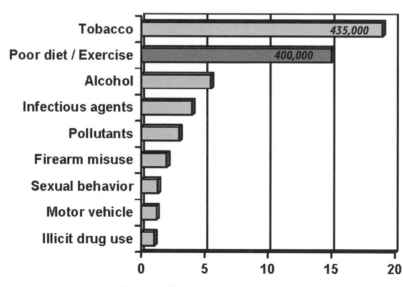

Percentages from scientific studies that attribute death to these causes

Percentages of all deaths source, CDC quoting from: McGinnis JM Foege WH. Actual causes of death in the United States. JAMA 1993. 270:2207-12 and (2) Mokdad AH, Marks JS, Stroup DF, Gerberding JL. Actual causes of death in the United States, 2000. JAMA 2004; 291(10): 1238-1246. Percentages used are composite approximations from published scientific studies that attribute death to these causes.

"Physical exercise is a physiological condition to which Growth Hormone multifunctionality is inextricably linked and is thus important physiologically and pathologically."
(*Growth hormone isoforms, segments/ fragments: Does a link exist with multifunctionality?*

Clin Chim Acta. 2005 Sep 8, De Palo, EF)

Degrees of health and fitness are often overlooked. We are a society with two health paradigms - sick and well. The paradigm of the "in between" sick and well, however, has been largely neglected.

Millions of Americans are one physician's visit away from being diagnosed with diabetes. Eight million Americans have undiagnosed diabetes, and 650,000 Americans will learn they have diabetes this year.

New government guidelines show that 23 million more Americans should be taking cholesterol medication to avoid potential heart attacks during the next 10 years (*National Cholesterol Education Program*, 2001).

The National Institutes of Health reports that 52 million Americans have cholesterol levels that exceed health recommendations. The cure: A medical prescription for exercise would be a wise national strategy.

Dr. JoAnne Owens-Nauslar, President of the American Alliance for Health, Physical Education, Recreation and Dance says, "We need to get people off their *buts.*" She explains, "I would exercise . . . *but*, I don't have time," and "I know I need to workout . . . *but*." Her message is clear and on target.

The New Fitness Paradigm

Is there a new and better way to think about improving fitness? *Yes!* This book is written to provide you with life-changing, energy-increasing, appearance-improving, timesaving fitness strategies, and a fitness plan designed for your age and current fitness level that will get results.

This book also provides you with extensive fitness improvement information that is supported by biomedical research – not the health and fitness gimmick of the month.

From fitness newcomer to advanced athlete, ***Ready, Set, GO! Synergy Fitness*** has a plan for you.

Richard Godfrey, a leading researcher in exercise-induced growth hormone from Brunel University reports:

> *A growing body of evidence suggests that higher intensity exercise is effective in eliciting beneficial health, well-being and training outcomes. In a great many cases, the impact of some of the deleterious effects of aging could be reduced if exercise focused on promoting exercise-induced growth hormone.*
> (*The exercise-induced growth hormone response in athletes*, Sports Med. 2003, Godfrey RJ).

This summary of the research concerning high-intensity exercise and exercise-induced growth hormone provides revolutionary insights for the future. It's simple; you have the ability to unleash one of the most powerful hormones known in science with a simple anaerobic workout.

Follow Richard Godfrey's research conclusion and his personal example:

> *I have been using the Ready, Set, Go! Sprint 8 Workout three times a week (usually on an exercise bike but sometimes running) and I have lost about 7 pounds in weight. I have noticed my recovery after almost every activity (even walking up two flights of stairs) has improved dramatically. I have also been able to use the energy boost this type of training has given me to get back into some 'proper' sports training.*

To start receiving the wonderful benefits produced by increasing this miraculous substance, finish reading the book first, then select one of the fitness plans in Chapter 11, implement the plan, and chart your progress.

You should see noticeable, even dramatic improvements in fitness, appearance, and energy during the initial eight-week commitment period. If you will make your fitness plan a priority for the next eight weeks, you'll begin to enjoy the benefits of fitness for a lifetime.

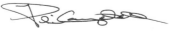

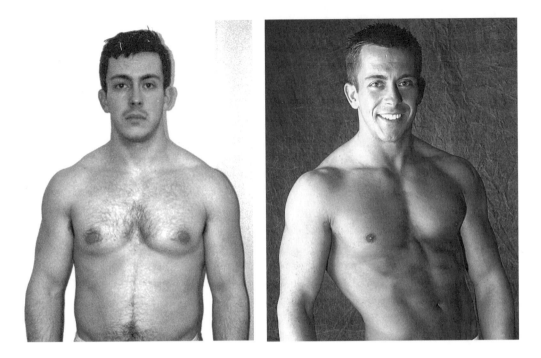

The **Ready, Set, Go!** program works! I was able to pile on new muscle faster than ever before while shedding body fat at an unprecedented rate. I'm now a personal fitness trainer, and I have all my clients do this program because it works, and it works for everyone. - **Alan White**

I've read your book twice now and I need to congratulate you on one of the best books available for understanding what really happens when you train. - **NASA Consultant, Jim Warren, President, Team America Health & Fitness, Inc.& Exer-Genie Training Systems**

1

Exercise-Induced Growth Hormone

Your body's ultimate fat-burning, muscle-toning and building, anti-aging, anti-middle-aging, synergistic agent

Human growth hormone is an extremely powerful substance that is produced by the body naturally. Some researchers consider it one of the most powerful hormones in the body.

Human growth hormone (frequently called HGH) is released in pulses - about twelve a day. And what it does to your body throughout life is nothing short of miraculous!

This is the substance that makes us, during childhood, grow several feet in height in just a few short years. After puberty, growth hormone begins to decline. Actually, it takes a nose dive until we reach the mid 30s, at which time the body begins to add body fat and some other not-so-positive things.

We joke about the weight gain that occurs in the early 30s and call it the "middle-age spread." But it's a real condition that medical researchers call the "somatopause."

The somatopause is related directly to the decline of growth hormone during aging. Symptoms of the sagging somatopause are body fat increases, muscle tone and size declines; good cholesterol goes down, bad cholesterol goes up, bone density begins to thin, and the skin begins to wrinkle.

"Human Growth Hormone is the most powerful anabolic stimulus known to science." (The Sports Nutrition Guide, Dr. Michael Colgan, 2002).

"The term 'somatopause' indicates the potential link between the age-related decline in growth hormone levels and changes in body composition, structural functions and metabolism which characterize aging. Physical exercise is an important environmental regulator..." (Aging, growth hormone and physical performance, 2003 Sep, J Endocrinol Invest., Lanfranco F).

Will the Real Fitness Hormone Please Stand Up?

For children, growth hormone is truly the "hormone of growth" as it was initially named by Dr. Harvey Cushing in 1912 because it makes children grow taller. Once we reach adulthood, however, growth hormone changes roles.

Growth hormone doesn't make adults "grow" after reaching their full height. Researchers show that when growth hormone is released during exercise, it targets and actually shrinks body fat for two hours after training. Whether it's called growth hormone, HGH, or the "fitness hormone," this substance can do some wonderful things when it's increased naturally in the body of a healthy adult.

New Landmark Research

When I completed the research phase for the first edition, the research was complete enough to draw hard conclusions about the type of fitness program that would make the body release growth hormone. However, the research didn't specifically test high-intensity sprints until later. Now we have more details.

In a 2002 study, researchers compared growth hormone produced by anaerobic exercise in several ways - resting (for a baseline measurement), after a 6-second cycle sprint, and after a 30-second cycle sprint.

SYNERGY FITNESS STRATEGY 1

Increase growth hormone naturally

The 6-second sprint method did move growth hormone some but didn't come close to the body's potential to release this powerful hormone. The 30-second, all-out effort sprint increased this hormone by 530 percent over resting baseline and 450 percent over the lesser intensity sprint.

Now we can conclude that it is possible to increase growth hormone by as much as 530 percent with this type of anaerobic exercise (*The time course of the human growth hormone response to a 6s and a 30s cycle ergometer sprint*, 2002, Stokes).

The researchers in this study also measured growth hormone for hours afterwards to see how long it stayed in the participant's bodies after exercise. This study confirmed the findings of earlier studies showing that growth hormone can circulate in the body for two hours after this type of exercise (*Impact of acute exercise intensity on pulsatile growth hormone release in men*, 2000, Pritzlaff).

Now we know that once exercise-induced growth hormone is released, this powerful hormone will target body fat like a heat-seeking missile for two hours after training. This is synergy! And it's where the "synergy" comes from in the book's title, *Ready, Set, Go! Synergy Fitness.*

New Research shows that one form of exercise can increase HGH by 530 percent over baseline. (The time course of the human growth hormone response to a 6s and 30s cycle ergometer sprint, 2002, Stokes).

Increasing exercise-induced growth hormone should become your top fitness goal. And step one is learning how HGH functions in your body.

"Exercise is a robust stimulus of GH secretion." (Growth Hormone Release During Acute and Chronic Aerobic and Resistance Exercise: Recent Findings, 2002, Wideman, L.).

"Intensity of exercise plays a key role in GH response to exercise." (Neuroendocrine control of GH release during acute aerobic exercise, 2003, J Endocrinol Invest, Weltman A).

What Does Sprinting Mean?

Sprinting is discussed throughout this book. Sprinting *does not necessarily mean running sprints.* The anaerobic sprinting workouts in the book can be performed in many ways - cycling, swimming, skiing, running, cross-country skiing, or even power walking. The workouts can also be performed indoors at home or in the gym on an elliptical unit, stationary cycle, recumbent bike, or treadmill. And since Vision Fitness (www.visionfitness.com) featured my Sprint 8 program in their award-winning, home cardio equipment, targeting exercise-induced growth hormone release at home is easier that ever!

Whatever the method of exercise, the goal is to reach all FOUR critical growth hormone release benchmarks with some type of exercise that is equal to the "winded" condition that most associate with running sprints.

How to Maximize HGH Release

There are some tricks-of-the-trade in maximizing exercise-induced growth hormone once it's released.

The gland that releases this hormone, the pituitary gland, is called the "master gland" because of its impact on so many other hormones. HGH may do more than you ever imagined. This hormone impacts every aspect of life and does so over an entire lifetime. HGH affects your career, appearance, self-image, ambition, energy, and performance - physically and mentally. Even relationships with family and friends are affected by this hormone.

Human growth hormone is stored in the pituitary gland until it is "released" into the blood system. (Beyond the somatopause: growth hormone deficiency in adults over the age of 60 years, 1996, Toogood).

Understanding how HGH functions will impact the way you think about exercise. And it may lead you to modify your diet, to add specific nutritional supplements, and perhaps even to change your sleeping habits.

The Somatopause
The Ultimate Baby-Boomer Bummer

It's been called the "middle-age spread" and the "middle-age bulge." But whatever it's called, it's a physical reality for 80 million middle-age adults.

Are you middle-age and experiencing weight-gain, energy decline, and loss of muscle? Are lab reports showing bad cholesterol going up and good cholesterol going down? These are all symptoms of the somatopause that typically begins in the 30s. Medical researchers report that the somatopause is related directly to the decline of growth hormone during aging.

It is characterized by high insulin levels and low plasma growth hormone levels, and how this leads to obesity, high cholesterol, and cardiovascular disease in both syndrome X and type 2 diabetes. (A reappraisal of the blood glucose homeostat which comprehensively explains the type 2 diabetes mellitus-syndrome X complex, 2003, Jun, J Physicol, Koeslag JH).

Growth Hormone
Declines During Aging

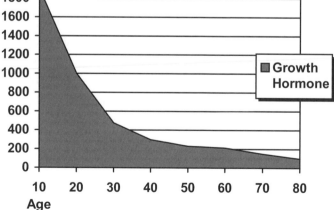

> *"Aging is accompanied by gradual but progressive reductions in the secretion of testosterone and growth hormone, and by alterations in body composition and functional capacity."*
>
> *(Neuroendocrine aging in men. Andropause and somatopause,* 2001, Endocrinol Metab Clin North Am. Anawalt BD).

Hormone Replacement?

Growth hormone replacement therapy via injections has proven successful in many anti-aging research studies. It has produced a 14 percent drop in body fat and an 8 percent gain in muscle. Researchers also report improvements in skin, bone density, and cholesterol.

These remarkable clinical results are not the best case outcome. These are the typical, average results. So, you can see why many are calling HGH therapy the fountain of youth.

Initially, HGH injections were given to children with clinical stature growth problems to help them grow normally. Today, there are 15,000 children being treated with growth hormone. And this therapy has proven to be very effective. For adults, however, there are better ways than injecting HGH to get the wonderful benefits of increasing this hormone.

Celebrity Anti-Aging Drug of Choice

It's widely reported that several well-known actors take HGH growth hormone injections for its anti-aging, youth-rejuvenating properties. HGH has been banned from athletes because of its ability to improve performance.

While there is research to show serious side effects are possible with this therapy, everyone knows instinctively that when you inject something into your bloodstream that costs $1,500 a month (that can put on muscle like steroids and pull 28 pounds of body fat off a 200-pound person), it doesn't take a rocket scientist to figure there's a price to pay in the long run.

There are better ways! Anaerobic exercise (as we've seen), adequate deep sleep, inexpensive supplements like 2-grams of L-glutamine before training will get the job done naturally!

The REAL Cure for the Middle-Age Somatopause

There are three cures for the middle-age somatopause - growth hormone injections (not recommended), a starvation diet (this doesn't work in a time-crunched, fast-food society), or the natural method, anaerobic exercise followed by a few simple fitness strategies to maximize exercise-induced growth hormone.

To be more specific, anaerobic exercise is the short-burst, get-you-out-of-breath quickly, sprinting types of exercise. You don't have to spend all day in the gym, jog for hours, or starve yourself. But it does require high-intensity exercise for short periods.

Now, before you go out and run, cycle, or swim a few full-speed 100-meter sprints or power-walk some steep hills, it's important to note that anaerobic exercise is the most productive form of exercise (from the HGH release standpoint), but it's also the most dangerous. Even young athletes need to warm-up and progressively build intensity levels or risk pulling a hamstring or tearing an Achilles.

Adults can successfully add anaerobic fitness training to their fitness program, but there needs to be a slow, progressive buildup period. Middle-age adults need to ease slowly into high-intensity anaerobic exercise.

For some reason, many of my X-jock friends believe that this warning does not apply to them. Even well-conditioned athletes, who can jog for miles, need a progressive, six- to eight-week buildup period.

It's a good idea to read Chapter 8, *The Sprint 8 - Targeting Exercise-Induced HGH,* and it's mandatory to get physician clearance before beginning a fitness program, particularly a high-intensity program like this.

"The fall in GH secretion seen with aging coincides with changes in body composition and lipid metabolism that are similar to those seen in adults with GH deficiency." (*Growth hormone - hormone replacement for the somatopause?* 2000, Horm Res. Savine R).

"*Moderate and light activities ... showed nonsignificant inverse associations* (for coronary heart disease risk)." (Physical activity and coronary heart disease in men: The Harvard Alumni Health Study. Circulation. 2000 Aug 29, Sesso HD).

High-Intensity is Missing

High-intensity, short-burst, sprinting types of anaerobic exercise is the missing ingredient in many fitness plans today. Yet this form of exercise is essential in getting all of the benefits the body has to offer those who make the decision to exercise.

Researchers show that high-intensity, anaerobic exercise plays the key role in increasing hormone release *(Meirleir, 1986)*. Researchers also show that increasing the intensity of training, *not adding more training volume*, will improve athletic performance.

We now know that high-intensity training improves athletic performance, and it also cures the somatopause for middle-age adults. So why is it that we quit doing anaerobic exercise typically before age 20? The long answer to this question is given throughout the book. The short answer is that we should never quit anaerobic exercise. Never. It should be a lifelong addition to our fitness plan.

When kids go out to play, do they methodically jog at the same pace for hours, or do they run, sprint, laugh, chase, zig-zag, climb, sweat, and get totally exhausted?

Here's another interesting question. When is the highest release stage of growth hormone during our life-span? It's when we are children - playing, running, and sprinting.

Slow-paced "cardio" is beneficial for burning calories and providing an endurance base, and it is a key element of every well-designed fitness plan, including this one. However, it's anaerobic exercise that takes us beyond the results of calorie-burning cardio by tapping into the most powerful body fat cutting substance known in science, exercise-induced growth hormone.

This book is not about quitting cardio. It's about adding anaerobic exercise to your fitness plan and multi-tasking it with cardio.

It was once thought that the buildup of lactic acid caused muscle soreness. Not true. Lactic acid is recycled in the body before soreness appears. Soreness is caused by numerous muscle micro-tears, or overstretching the muscle during exercise. (Delayed muscle soreness: the inflammatory response to muscle injury and its clinical implications, 1995, MacIntyre).

Leading Research

One of the most significant research studies concerning fitness training, anti-aging, and anti–middle aging was completed in 1999 by researchers at the University of Virginia School of Medicine.

Researchers there set out to determine the effects of exercise intensity on growth hormone release. They discovered that **HGH is released in the body in direct proportion to exercise intensity.** Simply, the higher the intensity, the higher the HGH release - once the HGH release benchmarks have been achieved *(Impact of acute exercise intensity on Pulsatile growth hormone release in men, 1999, Pritzlaff, Wideman, Weltman, Abbott, Gutgesell, Hartman, and Veldhuis).*

Once the research by this team becomes widely circulated and added to the textbooks in a few years, it will change the way the world thinks about exercise, fitness, health, and aging.

The "muscle burn" caused by the increase of lactic acid in muscles may be partly responsible for HGH release during anaerobic exercise. (Effect of acid-base balance on the growth hormone response to acute high-intensity cycle exercise, 1994, Gordon).

The Grand Prize of Fitness Training

Early research showed that a "particular threshold" of exercise intensity must be achieved before human growth hormone can be released *(Effect of low and high intensity exercise on circulating growth hormone in men, 1992, Felsing).* However, this "threshold" is evolving in the research to include four main benchmarks that must be achieved in order to release exercise-induced growth hormone.

You'll see this important information next. However, I can't overemphasize how essential it is for you to become an expert at understanding how to reach these four benchmarks during workouts.

"Growth hormone releasing hormone (GHRH) is one of the most important hormones in life." (Production and enhanced biological activity of a novel GHRH analog, 2004, April, Protein Expr Purif, Tang, SS).

Human Growth Hormone Release Benchmarks

Oxygen Debt

The out-of-breath condition resulting from high-intensity exercise during anaerobic training is an unmistakable HGH release benchmark. This is one of those conditions where "you'll know it when you've arrived."

Oxygen demand is an important regulator in the body's release of HGH during exercise (*Regulation of growth hormone during exercise by oxygen demand and availability*, 1987, Vanhelder).

Unlike other methods of fitness training, the goal of anaerobic exercise is actually to propel you into a winded state. The word *anaerobic* means "without oxygen."

After 8 to 10 seconds of 90 to 100 percent maximal high-intensity effort (like sprinting), or 20 to 30 seconds of 70 to 90 percent high-intensity anaerobic exercise (like hard intervals), the body experiences "oxygen debt."

During recovery from this state, the body pays back the oxygen debt by increasing the heart rate and supplying oxygen to the blood with hard, rapid breathing. And the **oxygen debt generated during exercise triggers HGH release.**

WARNING

Anaerobic exercise forces the heart muscle to pump fast and hard to pay back the oxygen debt caused by this form of exercise. See your physician before attempting anaerobic training. Even young athletes need to build up to anaerobic capacity.

Muscle Burn

The burning sensation that you feel in your muscles during exercise is caused by lactic acid. And reaching the "muscle burn" stage corresponds with release of HGH into your body. In fact, researchers show that HGH is released 16 minutes after reaching the "lactic acid threshold."

Lactic acid is a by-product of being "oxygen deficit" during high-intensity exercise. The lactic-acid-induced "muscle burn" is somewhat like a self-defense mechanism of the body. It lets you know that you're exercising anaerobically.

Reaching the "muscle burn" stage during fitness training is a noticeable sign that an important HGH release benchmark has been achieved.

HGH release occurs 16 minutes after reaching the muscle burn lactate threshold benchmark during exercise. (Growth hormone responses during intermittent weightlifting exercise in men, 1984, Vanhelder).

Increased Body Temperature

A third benchmark that must be reached to increase HGH is to turn up your body heat during fitness training.

Researchers show that increasing body temperature is an important HGH release benchmark (*Role of body temperature in exercise-induced growth hormone and prolactin release in non-trained and physically fit subjects, 2000, Vigas*).

Note: *A good warm-up should raise your body temperature by approximately one degree, and this is necessary for HGH release.*

Even in freezing temperatures, body heat can be raised by wearing adequate clothing. Don't let cold weather be an excuse not to exercise. There *are* temperatures, however, that will preclude HGH from being released. Use common sense. In most cases, however, working up a good "sweat" during training should accomplish this HGH release benchmark.

Researchers demonstrate that HGH will not release when exercise occurs in a cold room where body temperature cannot increase. (Characterization of growth hormone release in response to external heating: Comparison to exercise induced release, 1984 Christensen).

The increase of HGH during exercise is closely correlated with the release of adrenal hormones (adrenaline and norepinephrine). This occurs after reaching the "lactate threshold" benchmark.

(Threshold increases in plasma growth hormone in relation to plasma catecholamine and blood lactate concentration during progressive exercise in endurance-training athletes, 1996, Chwalbinski-Moneta).

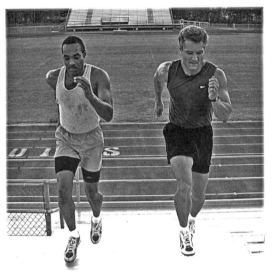

Running bleachers can reach HGH release benchmarks

Adrenal Response

The University of Virginia research team identified the "adrenal hormone release function" as possibly playing a central role in HGH release. The release of epinephrine (adrenaline) that boosts the body in stressful situations and norepinephrine, which maintains normal blood circulation, both play vital roles in HGH release.

Exercise must achieve the out-of-breath, slightly painful level of intensity that produces an epinephrine response before HGH is released.

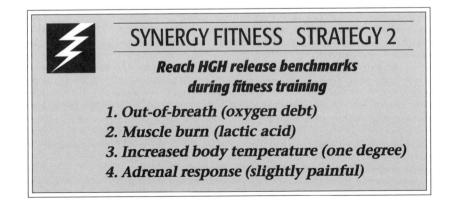

SYNERGY FITNESS STRATEGY 2

Reach HGH release benchmarks during fitness training

1. *Out-of-breath (oxygen debt)*
2. *Muscle burn (lactic acid)*
3. *Increased body temperature (one degree)*
4. *Adrenal response (slightly painful)*

Researchers show that the *physical age* of a person lessens the body's ability to release HGH. However, it's the *intensity* of exercise that is the key to releasing HGH.

In one study, young and old adults were tested for their ability to release norepinephrine during exercise. There was no statistical difference in performance at any age (*Young and old subjects matched for aerobic capacity have similar noradrenergic responses to exercise*, 1993, Kastello).

Timing of HGH Release

By the end of 20 minutes of high-intensity exercise, the body experiences a significant release of HGH. It continues to rise after the workout until it peaks approximately one hour into the recovery period.

After peaking, HGH slowly returns to baseline around two hours after training. One study shows that HGH will even last up to three hours (*Effects of blood pH and blood lactate on growth hormone, prolactin, and gonadotropin release after acute exercise in male volunteers*, 1997, Slias).

This means you have a two-hour, body fat burning "Synergy Window" open to you after every anaerobic workout that reaches the HGH release benchmarks.

Warm-up	Anaerobic Workout	Synergy Window

This is the "synergy" created by fitness training, and it's the "synergy" in *Synergy Fitness for Time-Crunched Adults*.

When you release HGH from exercise, you are turning your body into a powerful, fat-burning machine for at least two hours - that is, if you don't stop the release of HGH.

There are some things you can do to help . . . or hurt the release of HGH - before, during, and after exercise. These strategies are discussed next.

Growth hormone predominantly stimulated the turnover of free fatty acids in the recovery phase after exercise. (Exercise, hormones, and body temperature, regulation and action of GH during exercise, 2003, J Endocrinol Invest, Jorgensen JO).

Convert Energy to Synergy
During Exercise

Implement the following strategies before, during, and after fitness training, and you'll maximize exercise induced HGH release.

BEFORE Training

Don't - *Eat a high fat meal before exercise*

Researchers report that a high fat meal before training will stop the release of HGH (*Acute effects of high fat and high glucose meals on the growth hormone response to exercise*, 1993, Cappon).

High fat meals trigger an increase in a hormone called "somatostatin," which shuts down HGH. It is, therefore, important to limit any activity that increases somatostatin because of its negative impact on HGH release (*Chapter 2*).

Do - *Take 2-grams of L-glutamine before training*

L-glutamine is an inexpensive, single amino acid supplement that stimulates HGH release, and researchers show that 2-grams of glutamine will significantly increase HGH. Chapter 2 has more details.

Do - *Eat some carbohydrates to fuel intensity*

Researchers show that eating carbohydrates before exercise will help fuel workout intensity. Researchers report:

> *An important goal of the athlete's everyday diet is to provide the muscle with substrates to fuel the training program that will achieve optimal adaptation for performance enhancements* (Carbohydrates and fat for training and recovery, J Sports Science, 2004, Burke, Kiens, Ivy).

DURING Training
Do - Drink lots of Water

Researchers show that inadequate water intake during fitness training will "significantly" reduce the HGH response to exercise (*Effect of hydration on exercise-induced growth hormone response*, 2001, Peyreigne).

AFTER Training

Limit Sugar for Two Hours After Training

THIS IS THE TOUGH ONE! A high sugar meal after training, or even a recovery drink (containing high sugar) after training, may stop the benefits of exercise-induced HGH.

You can work out for hours, then eat a high sugar candy bar or have a high sugar energy drink, and this may shut down the synergistic benefits of HGH. Even before training, a high sugar meal will slightly impair HGH, but after training, consider your exercise-induced HGH release stopped dead in its tracks.

If you miss reaching HGH release during training (due to lack of intensity), you will still receive the calorie burning benefit from the workout. However, you'll miss the HGH "synergy bonus" of enhanced fat burning for two hours after training. This is an extremely important fact to remember if you want to cut body fat and shed a few pounds.

The University of Virginia research team demonstrated that carbohydrates are burned during exercise in direct proportion to the intensity of training. Fat burning is also correlated with intensity. However, **the actual fat burning takes place *after* the workout**, during the recovery.

This makes the "Synergy Window," the two-hour period after a workout, very important in maximizing exercise-induced growth hormone.

"We conclude that the exercise-induced GH response decreases when exercise is performed without fluid intake." (Effect of hydration on exercise-induced growth hormone response, 2001 Oct., Peyreigne C).

"We conclude that early intake of an oral protein supplement after resistance training is important for the development of hypertrophy (growth) *in skeletal muscle of elderly men in response to resistance training."* (Timing of postexercise protein intake is important for muscle hypertrophy with resistance training in elderly humans, 2001 Aug, J Physiol., Esmarck B).

"Despite the frequently expressed concern about adverse effects of high protein intake, there is no evidence that protein intakes in the range suggested (1.6 to 1.7 grams per kilogram of body weight for high intensity training) *will have adverse effects in healthy individuals."* (Effects of exercise on dietary protein requirements, 1998, Dec Int J Sport Nutr, Lemon PW).

Research shows that the intake of carbohydrates jump-starts protein synthesis, and the recovery process begins faster with carbohydrates. There are several studies involving young cyclists who compete for several days back-to-back, and quick recovery is their top priority, not maximizing HGH. If you're young and a quick recovery is your goal, a recovery drink with carbs and protein would be the best strategy. However, if you're middle-age, or need to lose some body fat, and want all the benefits from exercise-induced growth hormone, then apply the strategy of "limiting sugar for two hours."

Do - *Take 25 Grams of Protein after training*

While high fat meals before training and sugar afterwards limit the synergistic action of HGH, researchers have found that protein after training is beneficial (*Acute amino acids supplementation enhances pituitary responsiveness in athletes*, Di Luigi, 1999).

After training, protein utilization increases during the recovery period (Bilol, 1995). A high protein meal (with minimal concentrated sugar) or a protein supplement containing 25 grams of protein after fitness training is a wise muscle-toning and building, and body-fat-reducing strategy.

Protein supplements sold in large canisters with two scoops totaling approximately 25 to 40 grams is a convenient source of protein. One scoop of 25 grams is sufficient for most individuals.

The 25 Gram Protein List

Protein Supplement	1 scoop
Chicken / Fish / Beef	4 oz.
Nutritional Yeast	8 tbs.
Beef/Turkey Jerky	1 cup
Water-packed Tuna	6 oz.
Eggs	3

Specific details for high-intensity training protein needs can be found on page 62 in Chapter 2, *"Daily Protein Needs."* You can also find the latest research information on protein requirements for high-intensity fitness training and a free newsletter on the Web at http://www.readysetgofitness.com

An excellent resource is *The Sports Nutrition Guide* by Dr. Michael Colgan - www.colganinstitute.com.

Conclusion

To achieve the synergistic benefits of exercise-induced growth hormone, remember that you must first reach all four HGH release benchmarks during fitness training.

Once released, HGH will peak and remain in your body burning fat for two hours - if you maximize its release. To get the full synergy bonus available from exercise, implement Synergy Fitness Strategy 3 (below) before, during, and after every workout.

The next chapter, *Maximizing Exercise-Induced Growth Hormone*, will show you how to further enhance your body's ability to produce and maximize HGH.

"The response of muscle protein metabolism to a resistance exercise bout lasts for 24-48 hours; thus, the interaction between protein metabolism and any meals consumed in this period will determine the impact of the diet on muscle hypertrophy (growth)." (Exercise, protein metabolism, and muscle growth, 2001 Mar, Int J Sports Exerc Metab, Tipton).

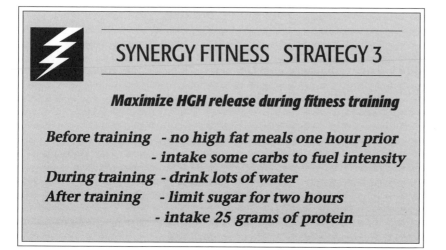

SYNERGY FITNESS STRATEGY 3

Maximize HGH release during fitness training

Before training - no high fat meals one hour prior
*   - intake some carbs to fuel intensity*
During training - drink lots of water
After training   - limit sugar for two hours
*   - intake 25 grams of protein*

I couldn't put it down. If you have reached a weight loss plateau, Phil Campbell's book may be exactly what you need to pump up your fitness routine. Even if you don't know the first thing about exercise, this book will help you map out a fitness plan. **Renee Kennedy, NutriCounter Health News**

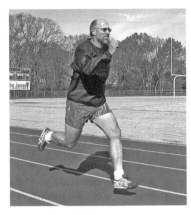

John Blankenship, 54, reduced his cholesterol 40 points with anaerobic training

Ready Set GO Fitness is perfect whether you are a beginner or an advanced athlete.
- Chris & Stacy Clark, Owners Powerhouse Gym Louisville, KY

Chris Clark, 48, Two-time NCAA, All-American javelin thrower, placed 8th in the world during the World Masters Track and Field Championships in Brisbane, Australia

Cutting calories is not always the best choice when deciding to lose weight. Sound nutrition with the addition of extra protein and an active lifestyle will increase your chance of dropping those unwanted pounds.
- Ron Nichols, LA Weight Loss

Phil Campbell takes the latest research in the biomedical disciplines of exercise science, medicine, nutrition, endocrinology and fitness for specific age groups, and presents a research supported system designed to improve the reader's health. Using his years of experience wisely, Phil is able to take complex medical subjects and make them understandable and practical.
- Cory Holly, Canada's Sports Nutrition Ambassador

2

Maximizing Exercise-Induced Growth Hormone

Enemy number one fighting your ability to maximize exercise-induced growth hormone during the two-hour *Synergy Window* is another hormone called "somatostatin."

Somatostatin regulates growth hormone like the thermostat in your home regulates temperature. This hormone will shut down exercise-induced growth hormone if some simple steps are not followed. From a fitness improvement standpoint, its important to do the things that increase growth hormone and not to do the things that increase somatostatin.

Essentially, anything common sense tells you is bad for your body may cause this hormone to be released. Examples - if you stay up all night, or if you're under tremendous stress, somatostatin may be released into your body, and it will shut down the benefits of growth hormone.

The number-one way to absolutely destroy exercise-induced growth hormone is to eat refined sugar after a workout. We'll get into the details of this topic during this chapter because there are several variables that come into play with this issue.

"We postulate that GH responses to strenuous exercise are only partially due to maximal GHRH activation. Next to complete inhibition of hypothalamic somatostatin activity."
(Involvement of endogenous growth hormone-releasing hormone (GHRH) in the exercise-related response of growth hormone, Int J Sports Med, 2003, de Vires).

"The Methuselah factor is contained within the pituitary system."

James Jamieson, pharmacologist and author,

Growth Hormone: Reversing the Aging Process Naturally. The Methuselah Factor, 1997). Methuselah was the longest living human in recorded history.

The hypothalamus gland (located just above the pituitary) controls the number of growth hormone (HGH) pulses and the amount that is released in each pulse. Your pituitary gland manufactures HGH. This pea-sized gland is located at the base of the brain about an inch behind the nose.

In normal individuals, the pituitary manufactures .4 to 1 mg of HGH per day. And it stores 5 to 10 mg. Individuals following high-intensity fitness plans are reported to manufacture and store even higher levels. This means that using every strategy available to increase HGH naturally will be beneficial.

Natural HGH Release Strategies

- Adequate "slow wave" sleep
- HGH enhancing nutritional supplements
- HGH secretagogues
- HGH releasing exercise

While HGH replacement therapy by injection is an appropriate treatment in certain situations, it's expensive and it has risks of serious side-effects. Clearly, HGH injections should be a "last resort," reserved for HGH-deficient individuals.

HGH injections take the place of the body's own natural HGH secretions, whereas exercise, diet, and sleep are natural.

Taking HGH secretagogues (sa-KREE-ta-gogs) is one strategy. This is similar to taking HGH-enhancing nutritional supplements. However, there may be a big difference.

HGH secretagogues can actually range from potent compounds of several amino acids and other protein transport agents to prescription medications. HGH-enhancing supplements are available over-the-counter at most nutrition stores.

"GH-releasing hormone (GHRH) and somatostatin are regarded as major regulators of this stimulation."

Acute Exercise has no Effect on Ghrelin Plasma Concentrations, J Horm Metab Res, 2004, Schmit A).

It's true that some HGH secretagogues can be derived from natural substances, and, therefore, rightfully wear the title of "natural." For the purpose of understanding HGH release strategies, however, a distinction must be made, for example, between "L-glutamine," an amino acid supplement, and the secretagogue, "symbiotropin."

HGH secretagogues may be a backup strategy if natural methods are not effective. But common sense tells us that it's wise to first give a full effort with the natural strategies of exercise, sleep, and nutritional supplements.

If you do not obtain reasonable results from the *Ready, Set, GO! Fitness* program and want to consider HGH secretagogues, I highly recommend reading James Jamieson's book, *Growth Hormone: Reversing Human Aging Naturally* (*Longevity News Network,* 1997).

Research at the University of Virginia demonstrates that exercise increases the frequency of HGH releases and the amount of HGH released per pulse/ secretion in a linear relationship to the intensity of exercise. (Impact of acute exercise intensity on pulsatile growth hormone release in men, 1999, Pritzlaff).

Side Effects of HGH Injections

Side effects of HGH injections in healthy individuals can be serious. They include acromegaly, a condition that causes short bones in the face, hands, and feet to grow unusually large. This condition leaves the individual with a "Neanderthal" appearance. This condition is permanent. However, increasing HGH naturally has been shown not to cause this condition.

Additionally, research on lab mice shows an increase in liver tumors when growth hormone is administered. When a mouse has a tumor, injected growth hormone appears to enhance tumor growth (*Overexpressed growth hormone [GH] synergistically promotes carcinogen-initiated liver tumor growth by promoting cellular proliferation in emerging hepatocellular neoplasms in female and male GH-transgenic mice*, 2001, Snibson).

Clearly, natural methods are the optimum way to receive the benefits of growth hormone.

It was not until the 1970s that we learned how the pituitary controlled HGH. Drs. Roger Guilleman, Andrew Schalyl and Rosalyn Yalow received the Nobel prize in 1977 for their HGH research. (NIH).

How Did HGH Become Famous?

Dr. Harvey Cushing officially discovered human growth hormone in 1912. He named it "the hormone of growth." Little happened until 1958, when Dr. Maurice Raben isolated HGH from human cadavers and injected it into a dwarf child. Miraculously, the child began to grow taller.

The time and effort involved in extracting HGH from human cadavers and animals - and the presence of mad cow disease detected in an early batch - slowed the use of HGH. The FDA approved synthetic (man-made) HGH in 1985. Protropin was the name given by Genentech for synthetic HGH, and it was exclusively used to treat dwarfism in children.

The annual cost of treatment is $12,000 per child. Today, 30,000 children are growing normally, due to the work of medical researchers. HGH injections for children with dwarfism are miraculous. Just talk to a parent of a child suffering from this condition who is now growing as normally as any other child.

The Rudman Experiment

Doctors seeking the answer to the following question made HGH famous. *Since synthetic HGH injections restore near normal growth in HGH-deficient children, would increasing HGH to youthful levels in older adults reverse the effects of aging?*

Dr. Daniel Rudman and colleagues conducted an experiment to answer this question. Their findings changed the course of medical research. In one of the most famous experiments in modern medicine, 12 healthy men - ages 61 to 80 - were injected with HGH three times a week for six months. The results were incredible. The injections restored HGH-deficient levels to youthful levels and subsequently reversed the effects of several years of aging.

An important point - the adults were instructed not to change their life-styles in any way so that the impact of HGH would be isolated during the study. The men gained 8.8 percent muscle mass, lost 14.4 percent body fat, and made age-reversing improvements in bone density and skin thickness.

Dr. Rudman and colleagues published their research findings in the *New England Journal of Medicine* July 5 ,1990. In their article, *Effects of human growth hormone in men over 60 years old.* The researchers concluded:

> *The findings in this study are consistent with the hypothesis that the decrease in lean body mass, the increase in adipose-tissue mass, and the thinning of the skin that occur in older men are caused in part by reduced activity of the growth hormone—IGF-1 axis, and can be restored in part by the administration of human growth hormone. The effects of six months of human growth hormone on lean body mass, adipose tissue mass, were equivalent in magnitude to the changes incurred during ten to twenty years of aging.*

New medical research taking place with HGH treatment is exciting, so exciting that the Growth Hormone Research Society has been formed.

Reported medical outcomes of HGH research are typically positive and call for additional study into new unexplored areas. Only one negative has emerged thus far, and it deals with HGH treatment of critically ill patients. Researchers report that HGH for critically ill patients actually increases mortality, prolongs ventilation, and increases the number of hospital intensive care days (*Increased mortalitY associated with growth hormone treatment in critically ill adults,* 1999, Takala).

Exercise is a potent stimulator of growth hormone (GH) secretion. This study provides evidence that the GH response to acute exercise may increase lipolysis during recovery. Lipolysis is the breakdown of fat stored in fat cells. (GH secretion in acute exercise may result in post-exercise lipolysis. 2005 Oct 4, Growth Horm IGF Res.Wee J

HGH Increases Good Cholesterol Cuts Bad Cholesterol

During one of the longest research studies on growth hormone - 10 years - researchers report:

> _Ten year GH therapy in adults with GH-D (GH-Deficiency) increases lean body and muscle mass, decreases carotid intima media thickness, and produces a less atherogenic lipid profile_ (lowers cholesterol).

Additional significant findings in this report are increases in energy levels and decreases in LDL cholesterol (bad cholesterol). HGH therapy also improves psychological well-being, researchers report:

> _The Nottingham Health Profile, used to assess psychological well-being, showed improvement in overall scores, energy levels, and emotional reaction in the GH-treated patients compared with the untreated patients_ (The effects of 10 years of recombinant growth hormone (GH) in adult GH-deficient patients, 1999, Gibney).

HGH Abuses

HGH is reported to be extremely popular with some elite athletes, bodybuilders, entertainment celebrities, and patients at anti-aging centers seeking age-reversing therapies.

HGH is currently undetectable as an illegal athletic performance improvement substance. Attempting to find a test to detect HGH abuse, researchers discovered that when a healthy adult injects HGH it suppresses the natural release of exercise-induced HGH for up to four days (Wallace, 2001, J Clin Endocrinol Metab). In other words, injecting HGH trains the pituitary to quit producing this hormone naturally for four days.

Filmmaker Oliver Stone, actor Nick Nolte, and actress Dixie Carter all acknowledge using HGH according to Ann Oldenburg, reporter for *USA Today* (November 14, 2000).

UPI-Washington reported that there may be as many as "500,000 otherwise healthy seniors getting injections of synthetic human growth hormone each year."

Now that injecting HGH has made the rounds in Hollywood and international athletic circles, it could move mainstream. Unfortunately, in the not too distant future, we may read that high school athletes are injecting HGH to enhance performance, to lose weight, and to improve appearance.

While injecting growth hormone does add additional HGH to the system, this causes an adverse effect of triggering the body to suppress its *own* production of HGH. And it's true; higher HGH levels will produce wonderful benefits through injections. However, there's a better (and much safer) way to achieve these benefits. Implement the strategies that follow.

Adopt the Synergy Fitness Strategy of Increasing HGH Naturally by:

(1) Commit to following a Strategic Fitness Plan - suited for your age, training experience, and current fitness level for an initial eight-week period.

(2) Follow a HGH-release enhancing diet - balanced diet / in moderation; high protein, low refined sugar, adequate carbs and fat, and nutritional supplements that are proven by research to stimulate HGH release.

(3) Get adequate deep sleep.

Melatonin supplements have been successful in treating sleep problems for shift work, jet lag, and some sleep disorders.

(Melatonin II: physiological and therapeutic effects, 2000, Bruls).

HGH is released during "Slow Wave" deep sleep

The largest release of HGH occurs during the first phases of "slow wave" deep sleep, about two hours into sleep (*Thirty-second sampling of plasma growth hormone in man: correlation with sleep stages,* 1991, Holl).

As we age, our sleep quality decreases, and so does the nighttime release of HGH. This decrease in HGH runs "directly parallel" to the decrease in slow wave sleep (*Age-related changes in slow wave sleep and REM sleep and relationship with growth hormone and cortisol levels in healthy men,* 2000, Van Cauter).

Adequate sleep is a critical HGH release strategy. In a similar study, researchers even suggest that there may be a future role for medicine to assist the night time release of HGH during slow wave sleep (*Interrelationships between growth hormone and sleep,* 2000, Van Cauter).

Dark conditions increase the natural increase of melatonin at night. Since adequate slow wave sleep is an important HGH release strategy, dark sleeping conditions may promote HGH release during sleep. (Secretion of growth hormone in patients with chronic fatigue, 1998, Berwaerts).

Melatonin Supplements Aid Sleep

Melatonin is a hormone that is made from eating protein, specifically the amino acid tryptophan - the most powerful regulator of the body's biological clock. Melatonin increases at night and decreases during the day in a light-dark cycle. During childhood, melatonin is released in higher levels, resulting in more slow wave deep sleep.

Melatonin supplements are inexpensive, widely used, and seemingly effective as sleep aids. In one year, 20 million Americans purchased melatonin supplements to self-treat their sleep problems. Some medical researchers feel that melatonin supplements are abused and have called for additional investigation concerning self-treatment of sleep disorders with this supplement (*Melatonin: aeromedical, toxicopharmacological, and analytical,* 1999, Sanders).

While melatonin seems to be an effective supplement, there are unanswered questions. Personally, I have tried melatonin supplements. They do make me sleep; however, I am sluggish the next day, and because of that, I don't like using them. Using melatonin for jet lag, for a night or two a year when needed, seems reasonable.

Some bodybuilders take melatonin supplements nightly in the hope of increasing their nighttime release of HGH. Excessive? Perhaps. The research is not conclusive.

How important is the HGH release during sleep? Researchers report that patients with chronic fatigue syndrome / fibromyalgia have significantly lower night secretion levels of HGH. Is there a relationship between chronic fatigue and HGH? There may be. And there's a great deal of research taking place in this area.

Researchers find that protein supplements improve muscle protein balance for middle age and elderly adults who use resistance training in their fitness plan. (The utility of resistance exercise training and amino acid supplementation for reversing age-associated decrements in muscle protein mass and function, 2000, Parise).

Protein During the Day
Aids Sleep at Night

A balanced diet with adequate protein during the day will help many get quality sleep at night - and in turn, assist HGH release at night. Most protein-rich foods (meat, chicken, fish) contain the amino acid tryptophan, which produces melatonin (for sleep).

Adequate protein during the day will allow your body to build up plenty of melatonin for natural sleep at night. And remember, high-intensity training increases the need for protein.

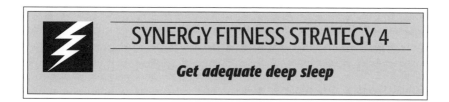

SYNERGY FITNESS STRATEGY 4
Get adequate deep sleep

"The current recommended intakes of protein for strength and endurance athletes are 1.6 to 1.7 g/kg and 1.2 to 1.4 g/kg per day, respectively." (What are the dietary protein requirements of physically active individuals, 2002, Jul-Aug, Nutr Clin Care, Fielding RA).

DAILY PROTEIN NEEDS INCREASE
For Endurance Training and Strength Training

Weight	Endurance Training*	Strength & Sprint Training**
100 lbs. (45.359 kg)	**54–63 grams**	**72–77 grams**
150 lbs. (68.039 kg)	**81–95 grams**	**108–115 grams**
200 lbs. (90.718 kg)	**108–127 grams**	**145–154 grams**

*Moderate-Intensity formula: 1.2 to 1.4 grams of protein per kilogram (kg) of body weight.
**High-Intensity formula: 1.6 to 1.7 grams per kilogram body weight.

An easy way to remember the daily protein requirement for high-intensity training:

Body weight X .75 = Daily Protein Requirement

"Increased dietary protein intake (as much as 1.6 grams of protein per kilogram per day) may enhance the hypertrophic (growth) *response to resistance exercise."* (Effects of exercise on senescent muscle., Clin Orthop, 2002, Evans WJ.

HGH Release Enhancing Supplements

Medical research about increasing HGH through nutritional supplements is rapidly advancing, but far from complete. Many studies have targeted amino acids as possible HGH-enhancing agents.

A few amino acid supplements boost HGH release in two different ways - by stimulating the release of HGH and by blocking the release of somatostatin.

The amino acid, L-glutamine, is successful in stimulating HGH release. And L-arginine is successful in enhancing HGH by blocking somatostatin.

Glutamine
World Champion HGH Supplement

L-glutamine is an inexpensive, single amino acid supplement that stimulates HGH. Glutamine also has a positive immune system function. Henry Mallek, author of *The Longevity Diet*, states:

> *The idea is to think nutrients. Instead of telling you to eat beans for protein, Mallek says, "think glutamine. That's because the principle anti-aging benefit of glutamine, found in beans, maintains a supply of antioxidants in the body.* (USA Today, Nov 14, 2000)

In *Growth Hormone: Reversing Human Aging Naturally*, author and pharmacologist James Jamieson cites research showing a 15 percent increase in HGH from glutamine supplementation. Jamieson's book provides an excellent survey of medical research regarding human growth hormone and an effective viewpoint of increasing HGH from a secretagogue release strategy.

A small dose of 2-grams of glutamine (typically two 1000 mg tablets) on an empty stomach with a carbonated drink will significantly increase HGH. Why carbonation? Jamieson theorizes that carbonation provides necessary "chaperone molecules," and this ensures that the glutamine gets to the right HGH pituitary receptors. Another report states that water is better than carbonation. However, the "chaperone theory" seems to have support in the literature. Hopefully, forthcoming research will clarify this question.

High-intensity fitness training can drop normal glutamine levels in the blood system by as much as 50 percent. This makes glutamine supplementation a wise pre-training strategy for several reasons.

A noteworthy research study at Louisiana State University shows that human growth hormone increases significantly 90 minutes after taking 2 grams of glutamine dissolved in cola. (Increased plasma bicarbonate and growth hormone after an oral glutamine load, 1995, Welbourne).

"Glutamine has a major impact on the functionality of the immune system." (Glutamine: recent developments in research on the clinical significance of glutamine, Curr Opin Clin Nutr Metab Care, 2004 Jan, Melis GC).

Glutamine does not produce a temperature-increasing "thermogenic boost" (like caffeine from a cup of coffee or the ephedrine boost from the herbs ma hung and guarana). Personally, at the end of a workout, I feel like I have extra stamina when I take 2-grams before training. And this allows me to train with more intensity at the end of the workout. Many readers have told me they also get the same effect from glutamine before training.

In one study, researchers report that after running a marathon, glutamine levels drop significantly, and this is the reason so many that compete in marathons get a common cold after the event (*Some aspects of the acute phase response after a marathon race, and the effects of glutamine supplementation*, 1997, Castell).

"Overtraining just prior to competition" is the standard answer given for the illness-after-the-event phenomenon, but Castell's conclusion regarding the glutamine drop appears to be the cause . Clearly, those who participate in high-intensity fitness training need to replenish nutrients used to generate energy during athletic competitions and training. Therefore, it may be a reasonable fitness strategy to consider supplementing with 2-grams of glutamine prior to training.

Pre-workout glutamine supplementation has also been shown by researchers to reduce the post-exercise decline in blood glutamine levels (*Effects of glutamine supplementation on exercise-induced changes in lymphocyte function*, 2001, Krzywkowski). So taking glutamine before training, rather than after, seems to have additional training benefits.

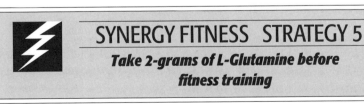

SYNERGY FITNESS STRATEGY 5
Take 2-grams of L-Glutamine before fitness training

NOTE: Glutamine has drug interactions with the chemotherapy drugs Taxol and Paclitaxel. Ask your doctor or pharmacist if you have questions. Also, GNC has an informative section on their Web site for checking drug interactions with nutrition supplements - www.gnc.com.

The National Library of Medicine has an excellent Web site at www.medlineplus.gov that you may find helpful for checking drug and supplement interactions. Click on the "Drug Information" link. This site has over 11 million citations from worldwide medical journals and is visited over 28 million times a month.

Another great resource is the Email newsletter produced by Dr. Gabe and Diana Mirkin; www.drmirkin.com.

Also, Chicago's Nicki Anderson is an excellent resource for diet and fitness information; www.RealityFitness.com. The Website for this book tracks research on L-glutamine and its role in HGH release; www.readysetgofitness.com.

Somatostatin is the hormone that acts in opposition to the positive HGH release in a thermostat type regulating function. (1996, Calabresi).

Arginine

The effect of L-arginine on the release of HGH was studied at the University of Virginia. Researchers concluded that arginine assists the positive HGH-releasing effect of exercise by limiting somatostatin release (*Synergy of L-Arginine and GHRP-2 stimulation of growth hormone in men and women: modulation by exercise, 2000, Wideman*).

One study successfully used 1.5-grams of arginine to enhance HGH by blocking somatostatin.

Large amounts of arginine have been used successfully with another amino acid, ornithine, to increase HGH release. Ornithine is manufactured in the body when arginine is used during the production of urea. These two amino acids may promote muscle building by increasing HGH and insulin. However, the amount of arginine used in the study, 13 grams, caused gastrointestinal problems.

"L-arginine may facilitate the effect of exercise by limiting somatostatin release." (Synergy of L-arginine and GHRP-2 stimulation of growth hormone in men and women: modulation by exercise, 2000, Wideman)

The bottom line on arginine as a viable HGH release agent is not complete. For example, one study from UCLA shows that arginine produces no increase in HGH with exercise and actually may impair HGH release during weight training (Oral *arginine does not stimulate basal or augment exercise-induced GH secretion in either young or old adults,* 1999, Marcell).

Arginine has no known drug interactions published at this time; however, arginine can inflame cold sores. Those using lysine for the treatment of cold sores (inflamed by stress and sun exposure) may not want to use arginine during the treatment phase because arginine can stimulate the virus that causes cold sores.

Arginine does have one noteworthy side effect. It produces nitric oxide (NO), a key amino acid used in herbal formula Viagra alternatives. You may want to keep this in mind the next time an herbal potency ad comes on TV - you may already have a key ingredient on your vitamin shelf.

New Kid on the Block - NO (Nitric Oxide)

Nitric Oxide (NO) was discussed at length in the first edition of this book because researchers reported that growth hormone assists in releasing nitric oxide (NO) to improve vascular health.

Researchers report: "GH, through its nitric oxide (NO)-releasing action, contributes to the maintenance of normal vascular...activity" (*Growth hormone, acromegaly, and heart failure: an intricate triangulation.* Clin Endocrinol (Oxf). 2003 Dec, Sacca L).

NO supplements containing L-arginine produce nitric oxide, which acts to relax smooth heart muscle and the walls of the arterioles so blood can flow easier.

Most everyone has heard about the effect nitroglycerine has on easing heart pain. In 1998, a Nobel Prize was awarded to Dr. Murad for discovering why nitoglycerine works - it increases nitric oxide (NO). The popular drug Viagra inhibits the breakdown of NO, and this increases its effectiveness.

Keep in mind that much of the science about NO supplements is new. While nitric oxide is shown to have many positives, too much of a good thing can be bad.

Researchers report that patients with chronic fatigue syndrome (CFS) have excessive nitric oxide (NO) production. "Elevated NO is known to induce vasodilation (widening of blood vessels), which may limit CFS patients to increase blood flow during exercise, and may even cause and enhance postexercise...problems" (*Chronic fatigue syndrome: intracellular immune deregulations as a possible etiology for abnormal exercise response.* Med Hypotheses, 2004, Nijs J).

Niacin

Niacin (vitamin B-3) assists in converting food to energy, making hormones, and lowering cholesterol. And niacin enhances HGH release by reducing fatty acids.

Niacin can cause "flushing" side effects, which I'm told are similar to hot flashes experienced during menopause.

Inositol hexanicotinate is a non-flushing form of niacin. And like niacin, it has been shown to reduce cholesterol.

Another form of non-flushing niacin is *niacinamide*. The Cooper Clinic reports, "niacinamide does not have the ability to lower cholesterol."

Large doses of niacin can cause side effects that range from flushing to major kidney problems (*Use of niacin in the prevention and management of hyperlipidemia*, 2001, Robinson).

Researchers report that the current World Health Organization recommendation concerning lysine should be three times higher. (Dietary lysine requirement of young adult males determined by oxidation of L-[1-13C] phenylalanine, 1993, Zello).

"It is concluded that an oral mixture of glycine, glutamine and niacin can enhance GH secretion in healthy middle-aged and elderly subjects." (Effects of an oral mixture containing glycine, glutamine and niacin on memory, GH and IGF-I secretion in middle-aged and elderly subjects, 2003 Oct, Nutr Neurosci, Arwert LI).

Deficiencies in niacin, folic acid, Vitamins B6 and B12, Vitamins C and E, iron and zinc closely mimic the damage caused by chemicals and radiation to DNA, and cause cancer.

(DNA damage from micronutrients deficiencies is likely to be a major cause of cancer, 2001, Ames).

Lysine

L-lysine is an essential amino acid and is famous for treating cold sores by interfering with the herpes simplex virus. By incorporating itself into many proteins, lysine acts as a partner with many other amino acids, particularly those involving nitrogen metabolism, calcium absorption, and amino acid involved in the promotion of growth and lean body mass.

Researchers at the University of Houston demonstrate that 1,500 milligrams of lysine and 1,500 milligrams of arginine immediately before exercise do not increase exercise-induced HGH. These supplements do, however, slightly increase HGH under normal, non-exercising activity (*Acute effect of amino acid ingestion and resistance exercise on plasma growth hormone concentration in young men,* Sumunski, 1997).

At this point, there's not a body of research to support using lysine or arginine as a HGH strategy.

Other supplements

Deficiencies in zinc, calcium, potassium, and other minerals significantly deter the release of HGH. The need for a good multi-mineral vitamin supplement for those who do high-intensity training is clear.

The quality of nutritional supplements is obviously important. We all know there are those who would make a quick buck selling poor quality supplements, if allowed. For example, some companies brag about the "USP symbol" placed on their product as if the product has been lab-certified for its high quality. This means that the pill has been tested to dissolve in your stomach.

Improvements are being made with supplement ratings. However, it is a good idea to stay with trusted name brands and trusted distributors when shopping for supplements.

Your Doctor Needs to Know

Nutritional supplements always need to be checked for side effects and drug interactions. Niacin (vitamin B-3) reacts with several popular medications, including oral contraceptives, medications to treat cholesterol - Mevacor and Zocor - and oral hypoglycemic agents prescribed for some individuals with Type II diabetes.

Thermogenic Weight Loss Supplements

Thermogenic supplements claim to increase metabolism and burn calories. These products increase heart rate and body heat, which, in turn, increase metabolism and calorie burning. However, there are side effects associated with supplements. The most famous thermogenic agent, ephedra, has been banned in the US.

A basic understanding of thermogenic supplements is important. These products can range from caffeine related products, like coffee, all the way to ephedra energy pills. The main problem with these products seems to be abuse and using them while getting overheated during the summer.

While ephedra supplements are prohibited, replacements will be created that increase body temperature to aid weight loss. Caution should be used with using any type of thermogenic supplement, especially on hot summer days.

NOTE: The purpose of this book is not to recommend nutritional products or their manufacturers. This information is intended to provide general information and is not intended to be product endorsement or medical advice. Decisions concerning nutritional products, health, and any health-related matter should involve consultation with the appropriate medical professional and your primary care provider.

"The US Food and Drug Administration has banned the sale of dietary supplements containing ephedra (ephedrine alkaloids) due to concerns over their cardiovascular effects, including increased blood pressure and irregular heart rhythm .... Effective on April 12, 2004." (Ephedra ban: no shortage of reasons. FDA Consum. 2004 Mar-Apr, Rados C).

HGH "Stacks"

HGH "stacks" are combinations of amino acids, vitamins, and herbs. The FDA does not regulate stacks as drugs, but as food. Typically, stacks include amino acids like glutamine, arginine, lysine, and ornithine, vitamins like niacin, and herbs like ginkgo biloba and barrenwort.

HGH Secretagogues

Considerable research is taking place with HGH secretagogues. This is the combination of several amino acids, the first being the development of GHRP-6 (six amino acids) in 1979 by Momany and Bowers at Tulane University.

These researchers led the way for extensive research into new methods of stimulating HGH release. These products are natural in that they are developed with *natural* amino acids. Secretagogues appear to be safer than HGH injections. However, they are also much more complex than single amino acid supplements like L-glutamine.

Research shows that an HGH secretagogue has positive immune enhancing qualities in the treatment of old mice with tumors and various cancer metastases. (Immune enhancing effect of a growth hormone secretagogue, 2001, Koo).

Research continues in this area, and emerging research has the potential for creating major discoveries in anti-aging, weight loss, and fitness improvement.

In *Growth Hormone: Reversing Human Aging Naturally*, James Jamieson recounts his personal involvement in the development of "Symbiotropin," an HGH-release agent. This compound utilizes L-dopa, a drug used in the treatment of Parkinson's disease, along with other amino acids.

If you are seriously considering HGH-replacement injections, you might want to consider experimenting with Secretagogues first. Why? HGH injections are substitutes for the real HGH produced by your own body.

Secretagogues on the other hand, act to stimulate your body to manufacture and release HGH. This is a huge difference with several ramifications. For example, growth hormone injections may actually train your pituitary to release less HGH.

I believe there are fitness plans available for every individual regardless of age, disability, and economic condition that will increase the body's production of HGH. However, there are other methods for those who choose not to exercise. It's important to note - there are side effects that need to be considered with every method of increasing HGH.

The current medical research concerning HGH secretagogues is summarized by Dr. Casabeill in *Growth hormone secretagogues: the clinical future* (1999):

> *The combined administration of GH releasing hormone plus GHRP-6, both at saturating doses, is currently the most powerful releaser of GH, devoid of side effects and convenient for the patient; it may also be an alternative to the insulin tolerance test for the diagnosis of GHD in adult patients. Their potential action at cardiovascular level is highly promising. Although the clinical future of GH releasing substances is appealing, probably the most relevant contribution has yet to be discovered.*

The final word on HGH secretagogues is not in yet. Therefore, it would be wise to check out the research before making a quick decision.

Insulin Balance

Researchers at the University of Milano, Milan, Italy, prove that too much insulin stunts HGH release. (Elevated insulin levels contribute to the reduced growth hormone (GH) response to GH-releasing hormone in obese subjects, 1999, Lanzi).

Insulin and growth hormone are interrelated. HGH does wonderful things for your body. However, the balance of insulin in your body can make or break the impact of exercise induced HGH release.

Insulin has several critical functions in addition to its well-known role of managing excessive sugar consumed in the diet. Insulin is important in controlling how the body uses fat (lipid metabolism), and it facilitates the entry of protein (amino acids) into muscle. And it may be the most important hormone in controlling energy during exercise. Some bodybuilders inject HGH and insulin to speed up muscle growth. Not only is this extreme. It's deadly.

There's a better way; anaerobic HGH releasing exercise, no sugar for two-hours after training, and a diet that is balanced and in moderation.

Without an adequate supply of insulin, the body's ability to filter dietary sugar from the blood is limited. When this condition first begins, researchers call it "insulin resistance." As this condition progresses, it may develop into diabetes.

Insulin Resistance
Making the body a body fat making factory

Individuals with high levels of body fat (usually 30 percent over ideal body weight) often develop a resistance to insulin. *"The heavier and more sedentary a patient is, the greater the degree of insulin resistance"* (*Syndrome X*, 2001, Reaven).

The body reacts to this condition by increasing circulating insulin to levels higher than normal. This not only interferes with HGH release but also it causes a cycle to occur that increases body fat even more.

When individuals with insulin resistance eat carbohydrates, normal processes are altered. Carbohydrates do not enter the muscle normally. They go back to the liver and are turned into fat (rather than being used for energy as they should be). The end result: more body fat and less energy.

"It is the high percentage of body fat relative to lean muscle weight that increases the cells' resistance to insulin," reports Nan Allison, licensed nutritionist and author of *Full & Fulfilled, The Science of Eating to Your Soul's Satisfaction;* www.AllisonandBeck.org.

Dr. Dave Unleashed newsletter is an excellent resource on this topic www.dedaveunleashed.blogspot.com. Dr. Dave Woynarowski's latest book, *The Immorality Edge* - www.telonauts.com - is a must read companion to this book as it discussess how Sprint 8 works at the cellular level to preserve the length of your telomeres. Researchers report, *"Our results indicate that telomeres length is preserved in healthy older adults who perform vigorous aerobic exercise and is positively related to maximal aerobic exercise capacity. This may represent a novel molecular mechanism underlying the "antiaging" effects of maintaining high aerobic fitness."* (Telomere length is preserved with aging in endurance exercise-trained adults and related to maximal aerobic capacity. Mech Ageing Dev. 2010, Larocca TJ).

"It is characterized by high insulin levels and low plasma growth hormone levels, and how this leads to obesity, high lipids, and cardiovascular disease in both syndrome X and type 2 diabetes." (A reappraisal of the blood glucose homeostat which comprehensively explains the type 2 diabetes mellitus-syndrome X complex, J Physicol, 2003, Jun 1, Koeslag JH).

The most severe cases of diabetes (Type I) representing 5 to 10 percent of diagnosed cases, are treated with insulin injections coupled with diet, exercise, and weight loss (CDC).

Refined Sugar is the Bad Guy

For a long time, we have known that we pay the price for eating heavy refined sugar such as candy and desserts on the calorie scale. But now we know that dietary sugar limits the synergistic impact of exercise induced HGH release.

If you are a lean, high school athlete, you can probably process the extra calories. However, as we age, without HGH to keep the fat burning metabolism synergized, body fat is increased and weight is gained all too easily.

Not only do high sugar desserts interfere with HGH, too much bread, cereal, crackers, and juice relative to the protein in the diet can have the same HGH halting results. People with insulin resistance are unable to process seemingly "normal" amounts of carbohydrates.

Please don't get me wrong, you need carbs in your diet to perform high-intensity exercise. Personally, I try to get some carbs before a workout. The key is moderation and timing. Don't let the craving for carbs after a workout stop the synergistic benefits of exercise induced HGH release.

If you're serious about improving health and fitness, rethinking the sugar in your diet is a wise strategy.

June Lay - www.junefit.com - offers an excellent Email newsletter that can provide additional motivation and information.

SYNERGY FITNESS STRATEGY 6

Maintain insulin balance with a balanced diet - in moderation

Exercise Improves Insulin Resistance

Resistance to insulin, as we have seen, occurs mostly in overweight individuals. This is a serious medical condition and is usually the first step toward diabetes, hypertension, high cholesterol, and cardiovascular disease.

Insulin resistance syndrome occurs long before these diseases appear. It occurs mostly in adults with abdominal obesity, general obesity, and family history. It also occurs in older adults who have lost muscular strength (*Insulin resistance syndrome*, 2001, Rao). This is why adults over age 90 have seen great results in clinical trials with weight training.

Researchers at Brigham and Women's Hospital in Boston measured the impact of being overweight (not obese, but merely overweight) on developing serious diseases. The researchers conclude that the risk for chronic diseases (heart disease, colon cancer, diabetes) is approximately twenty times higher for overweight people. The risks for serious diseases increase relative to the degree individuals are overweight (*Impact of overweight on the risk of developing common chronic diseases during a 10-year period*, 2001, Field).

Degrees of Health and Fitness

The following discussion concerning diabetes and hypoglycemia is directly related to sugar in the diet. The treatment for both of these conditions is the same - avoid sugar, lose body fat and add muscle.

Since many adults have not been diagnosed with either condition (yet), they "feel" they are operating within a healthy range. However, the absence of illness does not necessarily mean an individual is healthy.

"Insulin resistance can be improved by weight loss, balanced diet, and moderate-intensity exercise." (Insulin action after resistive training in insulin resistant older men and women, 2001, Ryan).

"There is compelling evidence that prevention of weight regain in formerly obese individuals requires 60-90 minutes of moderate intensity activity or lesser amounts of vigorous intensity activity." (How much physical activity is enough to prevent unhealthy weight gain? Outcome of the IASO 1st Stock Conference and consensus statement. Obes Rev. 2003 May, Saris WH).

Diabetes Resources:
The American
Diabetes
Association,
www.diabetes.org

National Institute of
Diabetes &
Digestive & Kidney
diseases,
www.niddk.nih.gov

Many middle-aged Americans may be closer than they think to being diagnosed with diabetes. There are 8 million undiagnosed cases today, and 650,000 Americans will learn they have diabetes this year.

Between the extremes of diabetes and hypoglycemia, there exists a state of *optimum wellness.* You should not be satisfied with resting at a level of borderline wellness when you can change course.

Rod Delmonico, former head coach of the University of Tennessee baseball team, says in his motivational speeches, *"Good is the enemy of best."* His point is clear; we should set our goals for optimum fitness and <u>not be satisfied with being absence of disease.</u>

Diabetes - A Disease of Middle Age

Diabetes is the seventh leading cause of death in the United States, and only half of the 16 million Americans with diabetes have been diagnosed. Untreated, diabetes can result in blindness; amputation of the toe, foot, or leg; kidney dialysis; and eventually, death.

The great news, however, is that most diabetics can be successfully treated with body fat loss, a sugar-free diet, and regular exercise. The Level One Fitness Plan in Chapter 11 is suitable as a starter program (with physician approval) for diabetic patients.

Diabetes Cure - Diet and Exercise

It is now an official U. S. government position that *Diet and Exercise Delay Type II Diabetes.* Health and Human Services Secretary Tommy Thompson made this announcement at the National Institutes of Health. The full report can be viewed at: <u>www.nlm.nih.gov/databases/alerts</u> <u>diabetes01.html.</u>

Insulin & Hypoglycemia

The symptoms of hypoglycemia are weakness, shakiness, anxiety, faintness, and personality & mood change. Because of the nature of these symptoms, hypoglycemia is often misdiagnosed as a mood/mental problem rather than a physiological problem - namely, low blood sugar. Hypoglycemia can occur as an overdose reaction to insulin injections.

A milder form of this disease, "reactive" hypoglycemia, can be spontaneously induced by stress mixed with a high dose of sugar. For example - someone on a fad starvation diet encounters a stressful situation and decides to blow the diet with a candy bar. Without protein or fat in the system, the pancreas shoots insulin into the bloodstream to counteract the sugar. The person gets giddy for a few moments and then begins to feel weak and even tremble. A diet lower in sugar and higher in protein typically controls the reactive form of hypoglycemia.

Achieving Insulin Balance for Optimum Fitness

Insulin balance is important not only to protect against the diseases caused by extreme insulin imbalances (diabetes and hypoglycemia) but also to achieve the highest degree of health and fitness possible.

The strategy for maintaining insulin balance is similar to the strategy of increasing HGH - balanced diet - in moderation (limited sugar), appropriate sleep, and productive exercise.

"Human growth hormone is reduced when insulin levels are elevated." (Elevated insulin levels contribute to the reduced human growth hormone response to GH-releasing hormone in obese subjects, 1999, Lanzi).

Many Americans who were thought to have acceptable levels of LDL, the artery-clogging "bad" cholesterol, are now considered to have excessive levels. (More people need cholesterol drugs, USA Today, May, 16, 2001).

Exercise Creates Synergy by Producing Antioxidant Benefits

High-intensity exercise not only increases HGH, it also has antioxidant benefits as well by scavenging the blood for free radical cells, which have been linked to cancer.

Some free radical cells are needed to fight disease and heal injury. However, when the body is exposed to environmental pollutants, free radicals are produced in excess. And it's the excessive free radicals cause damage and leave the body more susceptible to carcinogens.

Free radicals are also reported to have a role in heart disease and hardening of the arteries. The damage is actually done by the oxidation of free radicals. Oxidation in the blood operates in the same way that metal oxidizes (when left outside in the weather). When metal tarnishes, it is being oxidized. That is what excessive free radical reactions do in your bloodstream.

The traditional approach to combat free radicals has been to increase the amount of food rich in vitamins C, E, beta-carotene (orange fruit and vegetables—carrots, sweet potatoes), and selenium, and take antioxidant supplements.

Researchers report that aerobic and anaerobic exercise both produce small amounts of free radicals. (Remember that it is the "excessive" free radicals that do the damage.)

The free radicals produced during exercise "insults heart muscle." But this is actually positive because the "insult" causes the heart to develop an "adaptive response" that builds antioxidant defenses into heart muscle (*Physical exercise and antioxidant defenses in the heart,* 1999, Atalay). In other words, the heart muscle adapts, and becomes stronger.

Since high-intensity anaerobic exercise actually causes production of some free radicals to heal muscle tissue, I take a mega-dose of a vitamin-mineral supplement (mega-dose, not overdose) containing C, E, beta-carotene, and selenium in the mornings and again after a workout, or during the evening.

Like everything in health, fitness, diet, and nutrition, the keys to success are balance and moderation. New research from the department of Endocrinology at the University of Washington shows that antioxidant supplements actually block the clinical ability of niacin and a drug class called "statins" (simvastatin-niacin) to treat cholesterol problems (Cheung, 2001).

Don't rely on medications alone to keep you healthy. The research findings concerning statins were unexpected. Statins treat cholesterol problems for 12 million people. Many thought that they could continue to have poor eating habits, remain overweight, and operate without a fitness program by simply taking a pill (one of the statin drugs) to cover the damage caused by poor cholesterol numbers.

Now we see the Public Citizen's Health Research Group petitioning the Food and Drug Administration to add warnings for statins (Mevacor, Zocor, Lescol, and Lipitor) because of the risk of rhabdomyolysis (a rare condition that breaks down muscle tissue). Bayer even pulled its statin (Baycol) after 31 deaths from rhabdomyolysis *(FDA urged to beef up statin warning,* 2001).

On top of this bad news for individuals with cholesterol problems, *USA Today* reports that new government guidelines concerning cholesterol measurements mean that one in five adults should be taking medication for high cholesterol.

Is there any question that exercise should become a part of your lifestyle? Trying to stay healthy without exercise, and thinking that taking a pill will fix the problem only creates more problems.

High-intensity exercise that produces lactate may need to be considered "antioxidant agents" because of its ability to scavenge for oxygen (O2) free radicals. (Free radical scavenging and antioxidant effects of lactate ion: an in vitro study, 2000, Groussard).

Calculate the impact of your cholesterol values on your risk of a heart attack during the next 10 years at: http:// hin.nhlbi.nih.gov/ atpiii/ calculator.asp

This report means that there are 23 million more people who should be taking medications for cholesterol problems. However, new research shows that statins may have side effects. Another study shows that beneficial antioxidant supplements may block the effectiveness of the statins class of medication.

This research leads to two conclusions. (1) Don't rely solely on medications to keep you healthy. (2) Implement strategies that include adequate deep sleep, a *balanced diet - in moderation*, and a comprehensive fitness plan.

Stress Increases Somatostatin and Stops HGH Release

Stress causes many physical reactions in the body, including an increase in somatostatin. In one experiment, researchers administered drugs to stop somatostatin release in rats just prior to the onset of stress. The drugs restored the growth hormone that had been halted by stress.

Although the subjects of this study were rats, it can be safely concluded that high stress levels will stop HGH release with somatostatin *(Antiserum to somatostatin prevents stress-induced inhibition of growth hormone in the rat, 1976, Terry).*

Conclusion

There are several things you can do to help increase your body's release of HGH. The action plan below will help you implement these strategies.

THREE HEALTH STRATEGIES TO IMPLEMENT IMMEDIATELY

1. After reading this book, I will make the commitment to follow a Strategic Fitness Plan in Chapter 11.
    YES_____ NO_____

2. I will limit refined sugar in my diet.
    YES_____ NO_____

3. I will reorganize my sleeping conditions to increase deep sleep.
    YES_____ NO_____

4. I will make my physician a partner in my fitness improvement plan and ask for advice about any part of this book, should I have questions.
    YES_____ NO_____

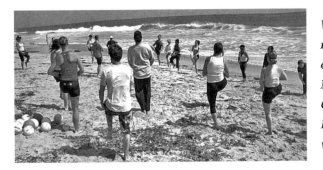

Warm-ups before running the Sprint 8 on the beach in Malibu, CA during Greta Blackburn's Fit Camp - www.FitCamp.com

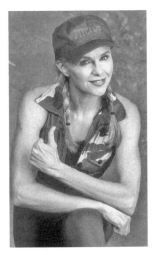

Ready, Set, Go! can take you to the next stage of fitness - regardless of your current fitness level.
- **Greta Blackburn, Editor, Ms. Fitness Magazine** Founder/Director of Greta Blackburn's FIT CAMPS, which take place in Malibu, Las Vegas, Mexico, Canada & Australia

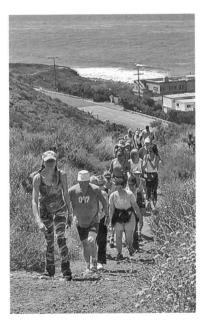

Greta Blackburn leading Fit Campers up THE HILL during her Fit Camp in Malibu, CA

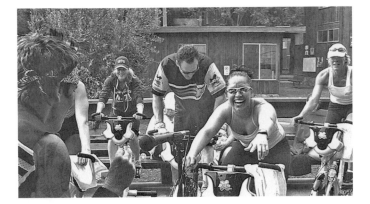

3

Redefining Age

Our mental image of how middle-age and older adults should look, act, and feel is extremely limiting and defeating. This mental image is deceiving millions into accepting a physical condition that's far below potential.

Bill and Jeanne Daprano of Atlanta, Georgia are redefining aging. They are what we should look like, act like, and feel like during aging.

At a recent master's track meet, I saw Bill Daprano run a strong 200-meter sprint in just over 30 seconds. Usain Bolt made the 200-meter event famous by setting a world record during the Olympics - that's great, but he's a young guy.

Bill is 76 years old in this photo. He looks much younger. From a distance, to see Bill run, you might say, "That's a fast high school or college athlete." He has set numerous World Records and two of them in the Pentathlon for his performance in five events (long jump, discus, 200-meter sprint, javelin, and the 1500 meters).

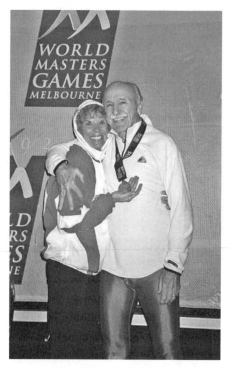

Bill Daprano is congratulated by his wife Jeanne after winning the gold in the Pentathlon 2002 Masters World Games

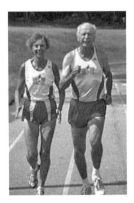

Bill Daprano receives the gold in the pentathlon during the 2002 World Masters Games. L- Silver, Fred O'Conner, Australia R- Bronze, Maurice Dauphet, Australia

The starting gun sounded as I was getting ready to throw the discus. I glanced and saw Bill take off from the starting blocks, and I watched him run as I always do at track meets for inspiration.

When he came out of the turn and headed into the straight way, he looked strong, young, and fast. I made the comment to 30 or so discus throwers, "That guy out in front is 76 years old." Everyone stopped in amazement to watch Bill run.

Bill running is art in motion! No painting has ever inspired me like watching Bill Daprano run.

Jeanne Daprano is also art in motion. She also holds numerous World Records. And they're in the tough, mid-distance races.

In the group, age 60-64 women, Jeanne set a world record in the 1500 meters (just short of a mile) in 5:46. That's four laps around the track minus 109 meters in less than six minutes! In another age bracket, the 65-69 women's group, Jeanne set another world record in 2002 by running 1500 meters in 5:48. This beat the former world record by nine seconds.

In 2009, Jeanne became the first 70-year old female to break the 7-minute mile mark.

Question: How many high school students can run 1500 meters in less than 6 minutes? Think about this for a moment. Here's a woman over the age of 66, and she can probably outrun 98 percent of all the high school students in the country in the mile.

Bill and Jeanne Daprano motivate me. They motivate me to get the message out that middle-age and older adults are cheating themselves out of the quality (and the quantity) of their life because they fail to get the benefits of fitness training.

Are you going to start the fitness program and stick with it? Only you can answer this question.

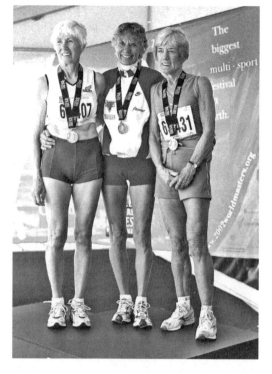

Jeanne Daprano receives the gold in the 400 meters during the 2002 Masters World Games. L- Silver , Margaret Peters, New Zealand, R- Bronze, Lorraine Woodman, Australia

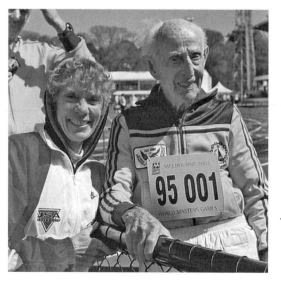

Jeanne Daprano congratulates Charlie Booth, age 99 after running the 100 in 28 seconds.

As I watched Bill finish his race, I thought of my dad, who died at 50 from a major heart attack. Bill and my dad would be about the same age. My dad missed 25 years of his life because he didn't have the health and fitness information we have today about how to perform high-intensity exercise.

He missed seeing three grandchildren born. Oh, how he would have loved my children. But that opportunity is gone. It doesn't have to be this way for you - if you'll make the decision today to add fitness training to your life, and keep it a priority for a lifetime.

Develop a Bill and Jeanne Daprano attitude. You'll understand what I mean when you read this - I asked Bill if he was going to the World Masters Championships (*different from the World Games*), and he told me that they aren't offering the five-event pentathlon, only the 10-event decathlon.

So what is Bill going to do, not go? Don't be silly! Bill told me that he is going to learn how to pole vault so he can compete in the decathlon.

This is the Bill and Jeanne Daprano attitude. Are you cheating yourself - and your family - from a Daprano full-of-energy life-style?

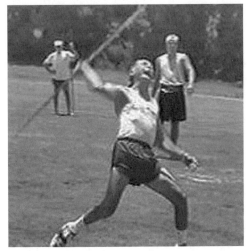

Bill Daprano setting the world record, age-group javelin throw

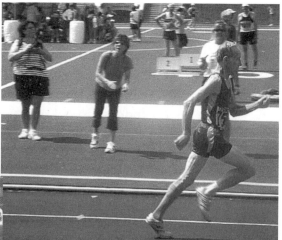

Christine Dewbre, Executive Director and Teresa Prinzo, Assistant Director of the Tennessee Senior Games encourage Charlie Baker (right) in the national finals of the 400 Meters

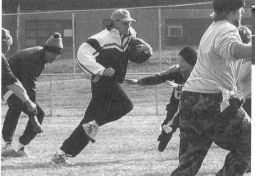

Terry Bumpus, age 53, getting an anaerobic workout playing flag football

Writer's Digest Review

Ready, Set, Go! Synergy Fitness for Time-Crunched Adults is a great title. In this day, most adults fall into the "time-crunched" category and are concerned with staying fit within their time limitations. I was hooked by the cover!

Phil Campbell's experience in the area of fitness is apparent. He has a tremendous amount of knowledge about the body and the effects of exercise on the body. His plan is outlined simply and reinforced by charts and tables. The exercises and weight training skills he suggests for the reader are outlined and illustrated with photographs. He uses models of all ages and fitness levels, which is an encouragement to the beginning fitness seeker. At the end of the book is a workbook section, allowing the reader the opportunity to put the plan into action with a minimum of thought. He or she can easily keep up with progress by using these charted pages.

The information is divided into small chunks, which help with understanding the relationship of the exercise to the body's metabolism.

The importance of using fast-twitch muscle fiber during exercise is reported in the *Journal of Applied Physiology* by Dr. Edward Coyle, Director of the prestigious Human Performance Laboratory at the University of Texas in Austin. Dr. Coyle, who is known for his work with Tour de France champion Lance Armstrong writes:

All-out sprint training especially stresses recruitment and adaptation of type II (i.e., fast twitch) muscle fibers that are remarkably and equally responsive as type I (i.e., slow twitch) muscle fibers in their ability to increase mitochondrial enzyme activity to high absolute levels. In fact, the low-intensity aerobic exercise that is typically prescribed for endurance training or health is not very effective at increasing aerobic enzyme activity in type II muscle fibers, which comprise approximately one-half of the fibers within the thigh (vastus) and calf (gastrocnemius) muscle in most people.

Thus low-intensity aerobic training is not a very effective or efficient method for maximizing aerobic adaptations in skeletal muscle because it generally does not recruit type II muscle fibers. The present report by Burgomaster et al. provides a reminder of the effectiveness of sprint interval training, performed three times per week, and it demonstrates that large increases in aerobic enzyme activity and aerobic performance capacity previously measured after 7–8 wk can occur after as little as 2 wk and only six sessions.

(J Appl Physiol 98: 1983–1984, 2005; doi:10.1152/japplphysiol.00215.2005. 8750-7587/05, http://www. jap.org 1983 on May 13, 2005)

4

Target Zone Training

If you are middle-age or older, or planning on becoming a fit, middle-age adult in the future, it's critical that you exercise and develop all three of your muscle fiber types - slow, fast, and super-fast. The reason is simple. It takes all three muscle fiber types, especially fast-twitch muscle fiber to perform anaerobic exercise. And it takes anaerobic exercise to release exercise-induced growth hormone.

If you're an athlete involved in a sport where running speed is important, then you'll also want to get the information in this chapter because it will help you learn how to develop the muscle fiber that makes you run fast.

Target Zone Training simply means that when exercising to develop a group of muscles, make sure you target all three muscle fiber types within that group of muscles.

Develop Fast-Twitch Muscle Fiber

You have three types of muscle fiber that make up your "muscles," and this is sometimes called *muscle composition*. The average person has approximately 60 percent fast-twitch muscle fiber and 40 percent slow-twitch fiber (type I).

There are two types of fast-twitch muscle fiber. The fast muscle (what many researchers call *IIa*) moves 5 times faster than the slow. And the super-fast (*IIx*) moves 10 times faster.

"Data suggest that changes in run training alter myocellular physiology via decreases in fiber size, Vo, and power of MHC I fibers and through increases in force per cross-sectional area of slow- and fast-twitch muscle fibers." (Single Muscle Fiber Contractile Properties During a Competitive Season in Male Runners. 2004 May 13. Am J Physiol Regul Integr Comp Physiol, Harber MP).

There can be swings in fiber composition. (*Muscle, Genes, and Athletic Performance*, September 2000, Scientific American, Jesper).

The following chart shows that while there are differences in muscle fiber composition, muscle types can be developed based on the way they are trained.

Muscle Fiber Composition

Muscle Fiber Types	Average person	Sprint trained	Endurance trained
SLOW type I	40%	40%	55%
FAST type IIa	50%	20%	40%
SUPER-FAST type IIx	10%	40%	5%

While we are born with slightly different muscle composition, the point is super-fast muscle can be developed if exercised properly.

Fast Muscle Crisis

When most finish high school (perhaps with the exception of a few that compete in college and the small number that make it to the pros), many become slow-twitch exercisers beginning at age 20. This is a mistake because muscle begins to waste away (atrophy) if it is not used.

Many adults continue developing slow muscle fiber with weight training and cardio at the gym, and with jogging. This typically only works slow muscle fiber. Most adults start the atrophy process of fast muscle fiber (the wasting away of muscle) on over half of their muscle fiber ... beginning at age 20!

No wonder we have an obesity epidemic. This year, 650,000 Americans will hear their physician say, "You have diabetes." The cure for the obesity crisis, the cure for the middle-age somatopause (the middle-age metabolism slow-down), the cure for insulin resistance and (in many cases) diabetes - is so simple that we keep missing it. The cure is natural. And it's free. Middle-age adults need to develop fast-muscle fiber so they can perform anaerobic exercise.

However, it can't be done overnight because the muscle fiber necessary to perform high-intensity anaerobic exercise has atrophied (wasted away).

You can build back your fast-twitch muscle fiber (starting slowly at first) by performing plyometrics to build the fast muscle (IIa fiber) and performing sprinting types of training to build the super-fast (IIx fiber) to the point where HGH growth hormone can be released through exercise.

Middle-age adults need to be doing more than exercising their slow fiber with strength training, cardio, and jogging. Don't neglect slow-muscle training, however; this is 40 percent of your muscle fiber, and, to a degree, it serves as a base for the development of the fast muscle fiber.

It's always recommended that you see your physician before beginning a fitness program. And even if you're in great condition, spend at least 6 to 8 weeks - slowly and progressively - building back fast and super-fast muscle fiber by adding plyometrics, E-Lifts, and sprinting types of training to your workouts.

Researchers show a direct correlation of HGH release with a wide variety of anaerobic and high-intensity aerobic exercise—from weightlifting to cycling, with fit and unfit men. There are "linear correlations" between GH release and "oxygen demand and availability." In short, you need to reach the out-of-breath stage to release HGH. (Regulation of growth hormone during exercise by oxygen demand and availability, 1987, Vanhelder).

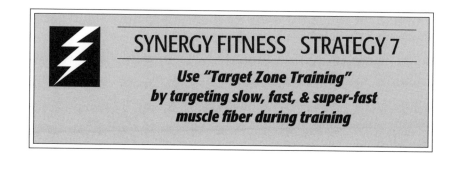

SYNERGY FITNESS STRATEGY 7

Use "Target Zone Training" by targeting slow, fast, & super-fast muscle fiber during training

Developing Slow Muscle Fiber

Type I muscle fibers are called **"slow-twitch"** because they contract slower than IIa and IIx muscles.

This muscle itself is red and is the main muscle group used in aerobic endurance training. Aerobic exercise like jogging, and walking, and the traditional methods of weightlifting, normally develops slow-twitch type I muscle.

> ## Slow-twitch muscles are in large supply in the body and are supplied with oxygen by many capillaries.

The "muscle burn" caused by the increase of lactic acid in muscles may be partly responsible for HGH release during anaerobic exercise. (Effect of acid-base balance on the growth hormone response to acute high-intensity cycle exercise, 1994, Gordon).

Developing Fast IIa Muscle Fiber

Type IIa fibers are called "fast oxidative" because these red muscles have a large amount of capillaries to supply them with blood. Type IIa is resistant to fatigue like slow-twitch muscle fiber. However, these muscle fibers move approximately 5 times faster than slow-twitch muscles. Type IIa fiber is used during moderate- to high-intensity exercise and matches with the exercise that targets the second gear–anaerobic lactate energy system.

Fitness programs targeting IIa muscle fiber would include interval training of 30 to 60 seconds. Some plyometrics, Olympic lifting, and E-Lifts (*Chapter 9*) target the IIa muscle fiber and may work the super fast IIx fast-twitch muscle.

Developing Super-fast IIx Muscle Fiber

Fast-twitch IIx (sometimes called IIb) is officially called "fast glycolytic" because it burns energy from stored glycogen for quick-burst. Type IIx muscle fiber aligns with the **first gear, ATP-PC energy system.**

Type IIx has relatively few capillaries to supply the muscle with blood (perhaps this is why the muscle is white). This super fast muscle fiber moves 10 times faster than slow-twitch. Exercising type IIx muscle fiber is critical in increasing HGH from exercise.

Researchers report "metabolic fuel" during fitness training (the way the body burns energy during exercise) and "tissue repair after exercise" play important roles in human growth hormone release. (Exercise and growth hormone: does one affect the other?" 1997, Roemmich).

Type IIx muscle specializes in scoring touchdowns, winning gold medals in the Olympics, delaying the middle-age somatopause, and reversing the effects of aging by 20 years.

The Strategic Fitness Plans in this book contain specific workouts aimed at the Target Zones in your body, which are your body's three muscle fiber types (within each body part).

With weight training, for example, the Target Zones are the three muscle fiber types (slow, fast, super-fast) within each body part. When you're working your chest, you should think about how to develop all three muscle fiber types in your chest. Traditional weightlifting only works the slow muscle fiber.

Without a comprehensive fitness plan that targets the three muscle fiber types, an individual could actually be exercising only half of the muscle fiber. "There was a significant increase in the proportion of type II fibers . . . Our results are encouraging in that they suggest an effect of human growth hormone on a specific aging-correlated deficit." (Growth hormone administration and exercise effects on muscle fiber type and diameter in moderately frail older people, 2001, Hennessey).

Creating Energy

The body has three energy systems that match the three muscle fiber types.

The three energy systems in the body operate somewhat like a car with three gears. **First gear** is called "ATP-PC." **Second gear** is "anaerobic lactate." And **third gear** is "aerobic." The body shifts to one of these three energy systems depending on the level of work or exercise intensity. Just like gas for your car, your body is fueled by energy produced by (1) your **diet** and (2) the **oxygen** you breathe.

Body's Energy Systems

(1) ATP-PC anaerobic energy system
Highest intensity level

(2) Lactate anaerobic energy system
Moderate to high intensity

(3) Aerobic energy system
Low to moderate intensity

An easy way to understand this process is to think of **carbohydrates and fats** in your diet as **firewood** and ATP as **fire**. ATP burns all its energy within 1 or 2 seconds and is refueled by the body in three different ways, depending on the intensity of the exercise.

It is important to note that ATP can only burn as energy when it has fuel to burn. **Oxygen** is a key source of fuel. When plenty of oxygen is available, aerobic processes continually supply fuel. However, when the exercise is one of high-intensity like sprinting, and there is not enough oxygen available for fuel, stored fuel sources can only make enough ATP to last for 6 to 8 seconds. This results in an **anaerobic** (without oxygen) condition. This is also a fundamental HGH release benchmark that you need to achieve during fitness training.

Running 150 meters to 400 meters (440 yards or one lap around the track) above 80 percent intensity will not only cause oxygen debt, but will also produce slight pain in the muscles. The body's reaction to the stress of anaerobic exercise may trigger adrenal involvement, which is also responsible for HGH release through secretion of adrenaline.

This level of intensity can be accomplished by exercise in the first two gears - ATP-PC, or the anaerobic lactate gear, but typically not in the aerobic gear.

Aerobic Energy System

When the body supplies energy aerobically - with a steady supply of oxygen in the blood fueling ATP (due to low-intensity exercise) - the *aerobic* system (**third** gear) is engaged. Carbs and fats supplying fuel for this energy system will eventually give out before the oxygen fuel source is depleted. Aerobic low-intensity walking, jogging, and swimming are examples of aerobic exercise.

Researchers show that lactic acid levels and corresponding HGH levels are "significant" in anaerobic exercise versus aerobic exercise (*Effects of anaerobic and aerobic exercise of equal duration and work expenditure on plasma growth hormone levels*, Vanhelder, 1984).

The exception is aerobic exercise that borderlines anaerobic and stays above the lactate threshold for 30 minutes. This level of intensity also stimulates HGH release (Wideman, 1999). An example would be a demanding 30-minute run at a 75 percent intensity level.

Zone In and Hit the Fiber Target

The following table outlines the alignment of muscle fiber types, the body's energy systems, and intensity levels. This table shows the type of fitness training that is required to zone-in on the target and work muscle fiber types while simultaneously hitting your body's three energy systems.

Targeting Muscle Types During Exercise

Target: Muscle Types	Super-fast IIx	Fast IIa	Slow type I
Energy systems	ATP-PC	Anaerobic Lactate	Aerobic
Speed	very fast	fast	slow
Capillaries	few	many	many
Muscle color	white	red	red
Oxygen capacity	low	medium	high
Zoning in: Types of training	anaerobic: Sprint 8 Workout	anaerobic: intervals E-Lifts plyometrics	aerobic: 20 - 30 minutes of cardio
Training Intensity	90 - 95%	75 - 90%	50 - 75%

Muscle Fiber Activation Process

The intensity of exercise determines the activation level of the three types of muscle fiber. During low-intensity exercise, the brain tells only the slow type I muscle fiber to respond to meet the demand. During moderate-intensity exercise, type IIa fast-twitch fiber responds to help once the nervous system senses that the slow fiber alone can't handle the higher intensity level. And during high-intensity exercise (like the Sprint 8), type IIx muscle fiber is recruited to provide movement for the exercise. This process occurs very quickly.

Researchers show that HGH release is tied to high-intensity exercise (*Chapters 1–3*). A comprehensive fitness improvement strategy should, therefore, include anaerobic (HGH-releasing) exercise as well as strength training, aerobic "cardio" work to build endurance, and flexibility training. The major components of a total fitness approach are discussed in the following chapter.

Conclusion

As you apply the principles of *Ready, Set, Go! Fitness* in your training, think about which muscle fiber type and which energy system is being developed with the type of exercise that you are performing.

If you think in terms of the muscle group and the muscle fiber within the group, you'll receive synergy plus from your training because you'll train the three muscle fiber types and you'll be training the three energy systems at the same time.

CONGRATULATIONS! You have successfully completed the *Ready* phase of *Ready, Set, GO!* The next section will get you *Set* and prepared for the action phase that begins in the *GO* section. The *Set* section contains a chapter for each of the major components of fitness training and an introductory chapter (coming up next) describing how to build your Strategic Fitness Plan.

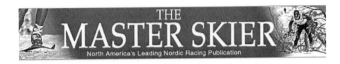
Book Review

Phil Campbell has done a very nice job in providing a practical fitness guide that "covers the bases" from balancing a fitness plan, to nutrition, to time constraints. Of note, we particularly liked his emphasis on quick, yet effective, workout models that have a great deal of promise for folks struggling to have enough time for workouts (who isn't?).

Another strong suit is the plethora of graphics and photos... particularly with stretching and strength exercises. It's also a nice touch to see Campbell use almost exclusively adults in these photos which may help "sell" the message that fitness is a lifelong pursuit!

Though not written specifically for XC skiing and/or racing, this is a resource worth looking into if you are in the market for a complete guide to fitness.
- **J.D. Downing, Editor xcskiworld.com**

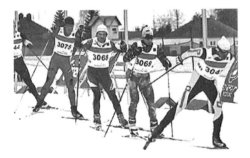

For more information on Masters XC Skiing, www.xcskiworld.com. The Master Skier Magazine published by Bob Gregg, & American Cross Country Skiers (AXCS) are excellent resources.

5

Building Your Fitness Plan

This Chapter begins the SET phase of Ready, Set, GO! It will show you how to build your fitness plan.

Your Strategic Fitness Plan will have five major areas of focus - flexibility, endurance, strength, power, and anaerobic training. Regardless of your age and current physical condition, your fitness plan should have planned workouts addressing all these areas.

If you're like me, there are some areas that are more enjoyable than others, but all are necessary.

The five areas do not need to be exercised daily. In fact, major muscle groups typically need 48 hours to recover. Overtraining can cause injury. And most injuries are actually "overuse injuries." Listen to your body and learn when to back-off and when to press-on.

The major components need training two times a week, and some components - endurance, flexibility, and anaerobic workouts - will need more frequent work.

The following chart outlines ideal training frequency by fitness component from the weekly perspective. This chart will give you a good idea of how the different workouts fit into a weekly training plan.

MAJOR COMPONENTS OF A STRATEGIC FITNESS PLAN

Fitness Plan Component:	Type of training	Time requirement	Training frequency	Fiber type	Energy system
Flexibility *Chapter 6*	Stretching	10 minutes	3-4 x week	All fiber	Aerobic
Endurance *Chapter 7*	Cardio	Target Heart rate for 20 minutes	2-3 x week *may be multi-tasked with anaerobic training*	Slow type I	Aerobic
Anaerobic *Chapter 8*	Sprint 8 Workout	20 minutes	2-3 x week	IIx	ATP-PC
Power *Chapter 9*	Plyometrics & E-Lifting	10 - 20 minutes	1 x week	IIa	Lactate
Strength *Chapter 10*	Weight training *Typical gym type of strength training*	30 - 60 minutes	3 - 4 x week	Slow type I	Aerobic

To get the full benefit of *Ready, Set, GO! Fitness* training, the benchmarks for HGH release - muscle burn (lactic acid), oxygen debt, elevated body temperature, and adrenal response (*Chapter 1*) need to occur on as many training days as possible.

NOTE: All components of *Ready, Set, GO! Fitness* are not designed to achieve HGH release. However, all fitness components are necessary. Flexibility and endurance training, for example, will typically not reach the HGH release threshold. However, without adequate flexibility and an energizing endurance base, it would be difficult, if not impossible, to perform anaerobic workouts that do increase HGH.

Specific workouts are illustrated in the following five chapters - one chapter for each major component of Ready Set Go Fitness.

For the anaerobic component, the "Sprint 8 Workout" is described, and the "10-Minute Stretching Routine" is recommended for the flexibility component. These workouts will be scheduled into weekly training plans programmed for the five different levels of fitness discussed in this chapter.

To illustrate how this works, the Level Two Strategic Fitness Plan for the first week of training will be used as the example on the following page.

For every Fitness Level (One through Five) there is a brief, highlighted, weekly plan. This weekly overview shows the training plan for a full week of comprehensive training.

"100 percent of the age-related decline in aerobic power among middle aged men occurring over 30 years was reversed by six months of endurance training." (A 30-year follow-up of the Dallas bed rest and training study: II. Effect of age on cardiovascular adaptation to exercise training, 2001, McGuire).

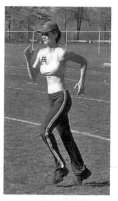

Cristi Doll, Ph.D. Clinical Nutrition and author of *The 10 Foods That Should Never Touch a Woman's Lips* running the Sprint 8

STRATEGIC FITNESS PLAN
Level Two

MONDAY	TUESDAY	WEDNESDAY	THURSDAY	FRIDAY	SATURDAY	SUNDAY
10-Minute Stretching Routine *Chapter 6*	**Weights** 1 hour *Chapter 10*		**10-Minute Stretching Routine**	**10-Minute Stretching Routine**	**Weights** 1 hour	Rest
Sprint 8 20 minutes *Chapter 8*	**Cardio-20** 20 minutes *Chapter 7*	*Make up day*	**Weights** 1 hour	**Sprint 8**		
				Plyometrics *Chapter 9*		**TOTAL WEEK TIME:** 4 hours
30 minutes	1 hour 20 minutes		1 hour 10 minutes	45 minutes	1 hour	45 mins

Workouts differ day by day in the training schedule to allow muscle groups adequate rest.

Wednesday is the planned make up day for Level Two. Should work interfere with your fitness plan during the week, you can use this day for catchup.

Notice the time allocation for the Level Two plan - less than 5 hours a week (and less than 3.5 hours for Level One). In the time it takes to play one round of golf or watch a couple of movies, you can complete a week of comprehensive fitness training that will dramatically improve your health, fitness, and appearance.

Get your week started right. Make Monday a good workout day. Mondays are the heaviest days in most gyms (no research on this, just a personal observation over 35 years). Mondays are hectic. But I've found that a good workout on Monday sets the pace for the entire week. Give Monday's workout your best effort, and the remainder of the week will fall into place!

Exercising at home is an effective method of training. (Effects of intermittent exercise and the use of home exercise equipment adherence, weight loss, and fitness in overweight women: A random trial, 1999, Jakicic).

In the time it takes to watch a couple of movies, you can complete a week of comprehensive fitness training that will dramatically improve your health, fitness and appearance.

Tracking Success with Training Logs

The Strategic Fitness Plan for your Level is also a Training Log for tracking your success.

By charting and writing fitness progress in your Training Log every workout, you can track your success and set goals for the following workout.

The keys for fitness training success are: (1) plan your work, (2) work your plan, and (3) record your results. Charting results with fitness training yields greater success. Your Training Log section (that's on the Fitness Plan page) contains a workbook section to record the amount of resistance (weight) used during weight training.

The Fitness Plans are designed to attack one day and one week at a time.

At the beginning of the week, plan your training schedule for the entire week. And before every workout, spend just a few minutes reviewing your performance from the previous workout and the plan for the day's workout. This will help get you mentally prepared and focused on what you need to get accomplished during the workout.

A sample of a completed Fitness Plan follows. This is what a completed Training Log should look like at the end of the first week of training.

NOTE: Pay close attention to the gray shaded areas on the Training Log. This is where you'll need to write the amount of weights used and the number of sets and reps that you perform during every workout.

STRATEGIC FITNESS PLAN

Training Log **Level Two** **Week 1** **Date_____**

Workout:	Training Plan:			M	T	W	Th	F	Sat	S
10-Minute Stretching	**3 x week (M, Th, F)** *Chapter 6*			X			X	X		
Cardio *Chapter 7*	**30 minutes 1 x week** *Tuesday or Thursday*				30 mins					
Sprint 8 *Chapter 8*	**20 minutes 2 x week** *30-50% speed/intensity during first 4 weeks. 8 reps 70 yards, walk back.*			6 70s				8 70s		
Plyometrics *Chapter 9*	**15 minutes 1 x week** *1 set plyo-drills at half-speed*							X		
Weight Training:	**Exercise:** *Chapter 10*	**Record Sets & Reps Performance** *sets/reps*		Record amount of weight used during sets in shaded areas. **NOTE: Perform E-Lifts** (Chp 9) on **push & press exercises**						
Chest	Bench press	2/12	2/12 2/12 2/10		100		105		105	
	Incline press	1/12	1/12 1/12 1/10		70		75		80	
	Chest stretch	30 sec	X X X							
Back	Pull downs	2/12	2/12 2/15 2/10		90		90		95	
	Up back stretch	30 sec	X X X							
Shoulders	Shoulder press	2/10	2/10 2/12 2/15		80		80		80	
	Front raises	1/10	1/10 1/10 1/14		12		15		15	
	Shrugs	1/20	1/10 1/20 1/20		20		20		25	
	Shoulder stretch	30 sec	X X X							
	Rotator cuff	1/15	1/10 1/12 1/15		15		15		15	
Biceps	Curls	2/10	2/12 2/15 2/10		15		15		15	
	Incline DB curl	1/10	1/10 1/12 1/12		15		15		15	
Triceps	Press downs	3/20	3/15 3/18 3/20		60		70		70	
Quads	Leg press	2/20	2/20 2/23 2/20		70		80		80	
	Leg ext	1/20	1/20 1/20 1/16		60		60		70	
Hamstrings	Leg curls	1/15	1/14 1/15 1/18		40		40		40	
Calves	3-way calf raises	1/21	1/21 1/21 1/21		100		100		100	
Abs	Leg raises	1/20	20 22 23							
	Crunches	1/25	25 25 25							
Obliques	Twists	1/20	20 20 20							

Age, Current Fitness Level & Training Experience Determine Starting Level

There are five levels built into the five Fitness Plans in Chapter 11. You need to place yourself in one of the five categories. When in doubt, place yourself in the lower level. You can always move up to the next level.

- **Level One** - newcomers, those not exercising regularly, adults over age 60, and children 14 and under.

- **Level Two** - adults who have been exercising, but not with comprehensive training or with high-intensity workouts, and adults age 30 to 70. There is some overlapping with ages due to variables in fitness levels.

- **Level Three** - physically fit individuals, at any age, who are active in a single aspect of fitness, such as distance running, weight training, or bodybuilding. Even for the experienced and physically fit, individuals entering at this Level need to keep in mind that new dimensions of training should be added incrementally. Listen to your body.

- **Level Four** - advanced physically fit individuals, ages 18 to 40, and experienced in high-intensity training.

- **Level Five** - advanced athletes.

Researchers report "vigorous activities" and "total physical activity" show the strongest reduction in coronary heart disease. Moderate and light activities are "nonsignificant" in reducing the risk of heart disease. (Physical activity and coronary heart disease in men: The Harvard Alumni Health Study, 2000, Sesso).

SYNERGY FITNESS STRATEGY 8

Use a comprehensive strategic fitness plan to increase flexibility, endurance, anaerobic capacity, strength, and power

Selecting Your *STARTING* FITNESS LEVEL

Fitness Plan:	Level One	Level Two	Level Three	Level Four	Level Five
Current Fitness Status	Inactive, just starting	Healthy, moderate fitness status	Fit	Very fit	Superb fitness status
Training Experience	Newcomer	Exercising some, but without intensity	Exercising regularly	Experienced	Advanced athlete
Age	Over 60 Under 14	30 - 70	18 - 50	18 - 40	18 - 30

What Time of Day to Train?

Researchers find that men at age 65 can achieve a hormonal response during training equal to younger men–if the exercise is similar in intensity.

(Hormonal responses to maximal and submaximal exercise in trained and untrained men of various ages, 1996, Silverman).

What's the best time for fitness training? This is a frequently asked question. Any time of day is okay as long as you get the job done . . . with intensity!

A recent study shows that time of day is not a factor in increasing HGH release during fitness training *(Cortisol and growth hormone response to exercise at different times of day, 2001, Kanaley).*

However, be careful not to train too late at night because this can impact sleep.

Fitness Training and Age

At any age, a comprehensive approach to improving fitness is clearly the correct approach. Otherwise, as much as 50 percent of muscle fiber in the body's muscle composition could remain untouched during training *(Chapter 4).*

As we age, activities that develop fast-twitch muscle fiber are typically dropped, and these muscle fibers decrease in size and strength. If fast-twitch fiber is not worked and developed during aging, fitness progress will be limited. Not using fast-twitch muscles during aging essentially means that these fibers (as much as 50 percent of the body's muscle fiber) will waste away through a process called "selective atrophy."

Since fast-twitch muscle fiber plays major roles in anaerobic exercise and increasing HGH, fast-twitch fiber development must become a priority.

Research at Tufts University demonstrates that adults, even up to the age of 96, can respond to resistance training and experience strength and muscle gains of up to 200 percent (_Exercise, nutrition, and aging_, 1992, Evans).

Older adults experience hormonal responses to exercise similar to their younger counterparts. However, it is extremely important for fast-twitch fiber to be maintained during aging. And this is done by following a comprehensive fitness plan that includes workouts targeted toward development of the three muscle fiber types.

For adults receiving growth hormone replacement therapy injections, unless prohibited, exercise should be included with their therapy. Researchers conducted a study with 35 adults with HGH deficiency and studied the impact of exercise in combination with HGH injections. The researchers show that future clinical trials involving HGH should have "planned exercise" as a part of the therapy (_Effects of growth hormone replacement on physical performance and body composition in GH deficient adults_, 1999, Rodriguez-Arnao).

In study after study, researchers conclude that exercise increases HGH release in young and old. Even to age 70 and beyond, high-intensity training increases HGH.

Researchers placed perimenopausal women into three categories—active, relatively active, and inactive—to determine the impact of exercise on the symptoms of menopause. "Significant differences" in the symptoms of irritability, forgetfulness, headache, and other symptoms were reported between the inactive and the two active groups. (The relationship between physical activity and perimenopause," 1999, Li).

Additional information about exercise and aging:

Medline, A service of the National Library of Medical Science
Toll free: 888-346-3656
www.nlm.nih.gov/hinfo.html

National Institute on Aging
Toll free: 800-222-2225
www.nih.gov/nia

Comprehensive Training for Bodybuilders

Many bodybuilders may only be working the slow-twitch muscle fiber with traditional forms of strength training that emphasize slow, squeezing repetitions.

This means that the super-fast (IIx) fiber and even the fast (IIa) fiber, which may represent half of their muscle fiber, may be untouched during training.

A tremendous opportunity for bodybuilders lies in the creation of a training plan that develops all the body's muscle fiber. Bodybuilders implementing Target Zone Training (*Chapter 4*), and working all the muscle fiber, might experience some extraordinary gains in muscle separation.

Shock Muscle Memory

Personal trainers, bodybuilders, and athletes experienced in resistance training understand muscle memory. They know the value of shocking muscles during workouts to pull out of a training plateau.

Researchers at the University of Canada investigated the effect of concurrent strength and endurance training on strength, endurance, endocrine hormone status, and muscle fiber. The findings from the 12-week study demonstrate that the combination of strength and endurance training yields a "significant increase in capillary development." And this research shows that "muscle memory" might be avoided with the combination of strength and endurance training (*Effect of concurrent strength and endurance training on skeletal muscle properties and hormone concentrations in humans*, 2000, Bell).

"Intensive exercise . . . is associated with higher HGH and testosterone levels, and exercise may have a role in counteracting the decline in HGH with aging." (Relationship of physical exercise and aging to growth hormone production, 1999, Hurel, National Library of Medicine).

Conclusion

Although all five major components of *Ready, Set, GO! Fitness* do not release growth hormone, however, all components are necessary.

Significant improvements in health, fitness, strength, flexibility, and appearance can be made with a commitment to train only four to five hours a week.

The building blocks of your Fitness Plan are contained in the following chapters. The five major components of fitness training each have a chapter that is ready to explain and illustrate exactly how to perform the exercises. The following chapters will also serve as future reference guides for the workouts. Should you encounter problems on an exercise, simply refer back to the chapter and the illustrations.

My son (a competitive cross country skier) told me about your book and I started the workouts following your basic approach. I am a 62 year old Orthopaedic Surgeon and run for cardiovascular fitness, weight control and enjoyment.

The Ready Set Go Fitness program has worked for me. I am running faster, have lost 5 pounds, have less muscle soreness than I had with just doing longer but slower paced runs - and enjoy my workouts much more. I have read a lot on fitness and the growth hormone rationale makes sense.

I have shared the book with my brother, a superb 70 year old athlete with a bad knee and it works for him on the bicycle and running up hills. I will keep recommending this approach as an integral part of an overall fitness program. - **Rolf Lulloff, MD**

I am truly amazed at the results in such a short period of time and I have just barely scratched the surface. I have lost about 15 lbs; my resting pulse rate has slowed 20% and I feel better physically and mentally. - **Wayne Key, retired chiropractor**

Stretching, no doubt is an integral part of fitness – and what a better source than Ready, Set, Go! Synergy Fitness. This program makes a lot of sense. A must for those looking for fat loss and long lasting energy. - **Namita Nayyar, President, Women Fitness**

I am noticeably stronger, faster, and more flexible since I implemented the Ready, Set, Go! plan. I hold author Phil Campbell directly responsible! I bought many copies of his book for family, friends and players and know I'm giving a valuable gift. - **Tom White, Publishing Consultant**

6

Flexibility Fundamentals

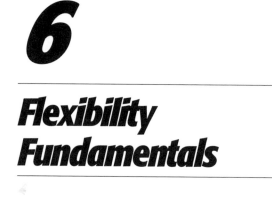

I don't like stretching! You heard me right. I have an entire chapter of my book dedicated to stretching, and I really need to like stretching. But I don't.

I'm naturally tight. And stretching is just down right painful. However, I said it in the first edition, and I'll repeat it again now. If I had to choose only one form of exercise, it would be stretching.

If you hate stretching, then you and I have a lot in common. But, you must, you simply must, add stretching to your fitness training. It only takes 10 minutes, four days a week. Just don't miss the many wonderful benefits produced by a regular stretching program.

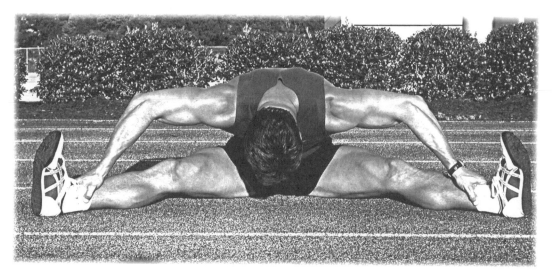

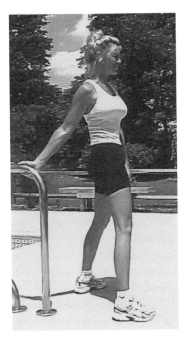

Stretching Does Not Release HGH

Stretching is not the kind of exercise that will release growth hormone, but it will prepare your body for the exercises that can.

Simply, if you don't have an appropriate stretching routine in your fitness program, you may be risking injury every time you perform anaerobic training like the Sprint 8 Workout or the explosive E-Lifts strength training.

New Research Reverses the Rule on Stretching

A three year old study about stretching is being cited in many articles today, and the conclusions reached by some writers may be harmful to your muscle, ligaments and joints. Stretching before fitness training and athletic training is being made out to be a time-waster, not needed, and even harmful. This is not true. In fact, there's a recent study that evaluates all the research on stretching, and the study concludes:

> *Due to the paucity, heterogeneity and poor quality of the available studies no definitive conclusions can be drawn as to the value of stretching for reducing the risk of exercise-related injury.*
> *(The efficacy of stretching for prevention of exercise-related injury: a systematic review of the literature, 2003, Weldon).*

Essentially, the researchers are telling us that there are not enough quality studies to draw hard conclusions about this issue.

The study that is generating all the hoopla was performed by the Kapooka Health Centre, New South Wales, Australia on 1,538 army recruits. It's a creditable study designed to show the occurrence of lower limb injury on a group of young army recruits. Despite what you may have heard about stretching before training, this is what the researchers report:

> *A typical muscle stretching protocol performed during preexercise warm-ups does not produce clinically meaningful reductions in risk of exercise-related injury in army recruits. Fitness may be an important, modifiable risk factor.* (*A randomized trial of preexercise stretching for prevention of lower-limb injury*, 2000, Pope)

The statement, "Fitness may be an important, modifiable risk factor" is very important. It simply means that age, weight, and conditioning of the study subjects may be an important factor in preventing or facilitating the injuries experienced in this study.

Three years after the Kapooka study, another study involving military recruits was conducted. The researchers in this study show that pre-training static stretching can prevent injury involving muscle but not joint or bone injury.

Researchers report, *Static stretching decreased the incidence of muscle-related injuries but did not prevent bone or joint injuries*, (Effect of static stretching on prevention of injuries for military recruits, 2003, Amako).

Based on the way some have written about this study, it's okay to run a 100 meter sprint full speed without stretching beforehand. Now, this may be possible for a small number of lean, young army recruits. However, does anyone believe that a powerful, muscled-up athlete or a middle-aged and older adult can go out and run a sprint - cold with no warm-up - without increased risk of injury? Don't think so... use common sense...and the full body of research!

Think about it; if an out-of-shape, untrained young army recruit performs high-intensity exercise, he may get injured, pre-stretched or not. And this is why researchers evaluating all the research on stretching conclude, "No definitive conclusions can be drawn..."

In short, there needs to be a body of research based on age, weight, conditioning, and the study needs to be performed functionally for the specific sport and type of exercise before life-changing conclusions are drawn.

The Truth about Stretching

New research shows that stretching can aid in the prevention of injury of stress fractures that plague distance runners. Researchers conclude;

Prevention of stress fractures is most effectively accomplished by increasing the level of exercise slowly, adequately warming up and stretching before exercise, and using cushioned insoles and appropriate footwear.
(*Common stress fractures*, 2003, Sanderlin)

Stretching offers many benefits. Researchers show that prolonged stretching (in the form of yoga) with moderate aerobic exercise and diet control will reduce cholesterol and significantly reverse hardening of the arteries (20 percent regression) in adults with proven coronary atherosclerotic disease. After one year in a yoga program, participants lost weight, reduced cholesterol, and improved their exercise capacity, (*Retardation of coronary atherosclerosis with yoga lifestyle intervention*, 2000, Manchanda).

Stretching offers many benefits, but there is an issue about the type of stretching and the timing of stretching before training and athletic competitions.

Use Dynamic Stretching Before Games and Practice

There are several hybrid forms of stretching, however there are two main types of stretching, static (holding a stretching exercise in one position without movement) and dynamic stretching, which means moving while stretching (arm swings, knee rotations, neck circles).

Researchers show that athletes should not perform prolonged static stretching before the big game or a key practice session because this slows muscle activation for around an hour afterwards, (*Reduced strength after passive stretch of the human plantar flexors*, 2000, Fowles).

Using dynamic stretching is a wise pre-competition strategy. Static stretching builds flexibility and should be performed regularly, just not immediately before a big game or a key practice session.

Warming up prior to a high-intensity, ballistic, athletic event is an absolute rule - never to be broken, and stretching can be combined (multi-tasked) as part of the warm-up. The goal of the warm-up is to get the blood flowing and raise body temperature (one degree) prior to athletic competitions and high-intensity training.

It's desirable to have the athlete's muscle, ligaments, and joints experience the range of motion required of the sport during the warm-up.

> *"Prolonged" stretching decreases strength for up to an hour after stretching by slightly impairing muscle activation.* (Reduced strength after passive stretch of the human plantar flexors, 2000, Fowles).

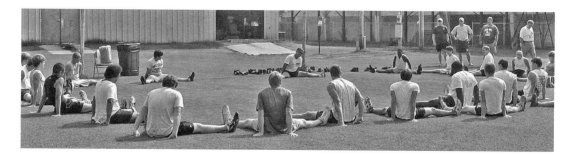

Use Static Stretching
After or Away from Practice

Gains in flexibility are dependent on the "duration" of stretch-hold position, and researchers show the best "stretch-hold position" (for time-spent) to increase flexibility is 30 seconds. (*The effect of time on static stretch on the flexibility of the hamstring muscles*, 1994, Bandy). "Best" means optimal results for time-spent. You can get positive results with 2 minute stretch-holds, but 30 seconds yields equal results.

This type of stretching is positive for athletes and adults of all ages. Researchers show in one study that longer hold stretching positions are of great benefit for adults over age 65:

Longer hold times during stretching of the hamstring muscles resulted in a greater rate of gains in range of motion (ROM) and a more sustained increase in ROM in elderly subjects. (*The effect of duration of stretching of the hamstring muscle group for increasing range of motion in people aged 65 years or older*, 2001, Feland).

Adults ages 21 to 45 with tight hamstrings also get the best results from static stretching with 30-second stretch-hold positions. Researchers report that static stretching is two times more effective than dynamic range of motion (DROM) for this group of non-competitive athletes. Researchers report;

The results of this study suggest that, although both static stretch and DROM (dynamic stretching) will increase hamstring flexibility, a 30-second static stretch was more effective than the newer technique," DROM, *for enhancing flexibility.* (*The effect of static stretch and dynamic range of motion training on the flexibility of the hamstring muscles*, 2001, Bandy).

Keep in mind there are important lessons in these studies, but the studies apply to a specific age group (over 65, and ages

21 - 45,) and a specific physical condition (tight hamstrings). If we apply the results of a study with these variables to young athletes, we may be wrong.

While it's reasonable to conclude (as I have for training purposes) that static stretching away from practice is an effective strategy for adults with tight hamstrings, this study doesn't specifically prove that point. It's clearly a mistake to take the findings of one study and create an absolute fact. Look at the whole body of research about a topic before making a life-changing training decision.

The 10-Minute Stretching Routine

The stretching routine illustrated in this chapter is recommended for all ages and fitness levels. The 10-Minute Stretching Routine is programmed into every Fitness Plan in this book - typically for four days a week. This stretching routine should be performed more frequently than other forms of training that require longer recovery periods.

All stretching positions in the 10-Minute Stretching Routine are static, which means there should be no bouncing. Slowly move into the illustrated stretching position and get "fully stretched." You will know when you are fully stretched when you "feel the limit" (because you can't go any further). Again, once you get into the stretch-hold position, **DO NOT BOUNCE**, as this can cause injury. And always move in "slow motion" while stretching.

You should feel slight discomfort but no sharp pain. Remain in the stretch-hold position for 30 seconds (without bouncing), and then, very slowly, ease out of the position before going to the next stretching position. The stretching positions in the 10-Minute Stretching Routine impact most major muscle groups, except chest, shoulders, and upper back. For time saving through multi-tasking exercises, upper-body stretching is to be performed during weight training.

1. Hamstring Stretch

Sitting on the floor with one leg extended, toes up, and the other leg bent, slowly pull forward. You will feel this in the target area - hamstrings, calves, and lower back.

Once in the fully stretched position (there should be slight discomfort, but no pain), remain in the stretch-hold position for 30 seconds. Then, slowly, ease out of the position.

On cold days, or days when you feel less flexible, you may want to repeat the 30-second stretch-hold position two times before switching legs. Yoga practitioners sometimes call this the "Head To Knee" pose. A pose, in yoga terms, means stretching position.

Almost every muscle group receives benefit from this stretching position - hamstrings, calves, Achilles tendons, groin, quadriceps (quads), obliques, shoulders, upper and lower back. This is a key stretching position and serves as a warm-up for the other stretching positions that follow.

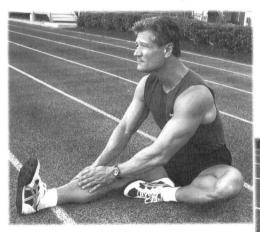

Start

Photographs by Holly Campbell

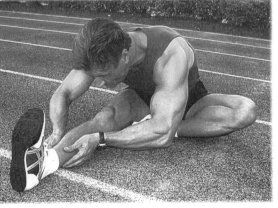

Pull forward
position

As human beings, we live life on concrete. Just think about how many hours a day you spend on hard surfaces. We adapt by wearing nice, cushioned shoes with elevated padded heels. This allows us to handle hard surfaces, but it also tightens muscles and tendons in the legs. To a degree, the lower back, Achilles, calves and hamstrings are being trained daily to become tight. And it takes stretching these muscles groups just to get even.

When the hamstrings are flexible, this typically helps the other related muscle groups that need flexibility. Concerning hamstring flexibility, researchers report:

> *A significant increase in hamstring length can be maintained for up to 24 hours when using static stretching. Muscle length gains are greatest immediately after stretching and decline within 15 minutes. The addition of a warm-up exercise prior to stretching does not appear to significantly increase the effectiveness of static hamstring stretching.*
> (The effect of static stretch and warm-up exercise, 2003 Dec, Orthop Sports Phys Ther, de Weijer).

"The results of this study suggest that a duration of 30 seconds is an effective time of stretching for enhancing the flexibility of the hamstring muscles. Given the information that no increase in flexibility of the hamstring muscles occurred by increasing the duration of stretching from 30 to 60 seconds, the use of the longer duration of stretching for an acute effect must be questioned."
(The effect of time on static stretch on the flexibility of the hamstring muscles, 1994 Mar, Phys Ther, Bandy WD).

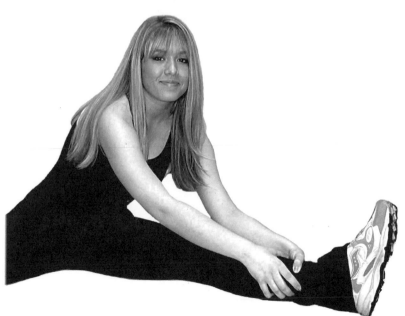

Holly Campbell stretching hamstrings

2. Torso Twist

The move from the Hamstring Stretch to the Torso Twist position is easy. Keep the right leg straight, toes up, and take the left leg and cross it over the right leg as shown below by Christine Campbell. Place the left foot above the knee.

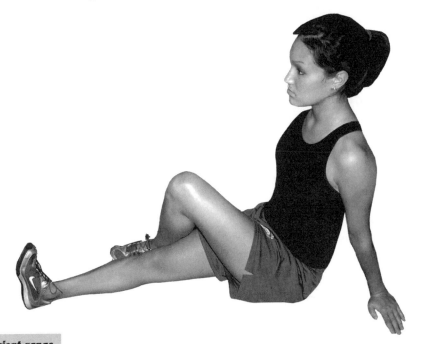

"Insufficient range of motion at the hip throws considerable stress on the other lower limb segments." (Prevention of hip and knee injuries in ballet dancers, Sports Med, 1988 Nov, Reid DC).

This stretching position targets the lower back, shoulders, lats, traps, hips, groin, gluts, obliques (love handles), and even the neck will feel the stretch of this position.

Moving in slow motion, place the right arm over the left knee and push against the knee while twisting the torso to the left. You should feel the stretch in the targeted areas; hips torso, shoulders, and neck. To maximize the effectiveness of this stretching position, try to twist your head as far to the left as possible.

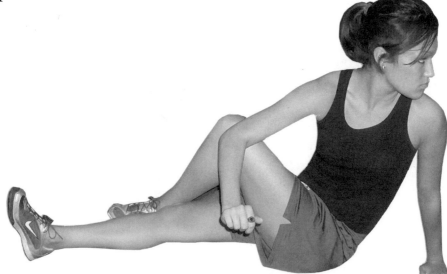

After holding this stretch for 30 seconds, slowly ease out of the position, switch legs, and repeat on the other side.

Doing this stretching program four times a week will increase your range of motion in several areas, and your gains in flexibility should become noticeable in a few weeks.

You can easily measure your improvement in flexibility with the *sit-and-reach test*, which is performed by sitting with both legs extended forward with knees locked. Now, reach with both arms and see how many inches you can reach beyond your toes (with knees locked). It's a good idea to self-measure your flexibility every week initially so you will be rewarded for your effort with measurable improvement.

Typically, athletes attending my Speed Camps will see flexibility gains of four inches in 30 days with this routine.

3. Hamstring Leg-Raise Stretch

The Hamstring Leg-Raise Stretch can be a difficult stretching position initially. While lying on your back, raise your right leg and with your right hand, grab your ankle (or your sock, pant leg, or place your hand behind-your-knee).

Straighten your leg and hold for 30 seconds in the fully stretched position as shown. Repeat with the other leg.

The advanced version is to place the left hand on the right ankle.

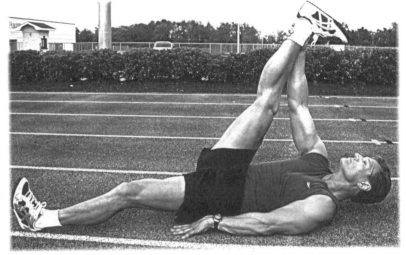

4. Knee-Hug Stretch

The Knee-Hug Stretch is an easy move from the Leg-Raise Stretch. Simply lower the leg and pull the knee into the chest with both hands, hold for 30 seconds. Repeat on the other side.

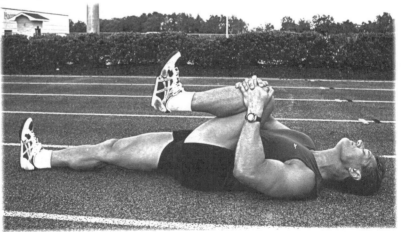

Knee Hug Stretch

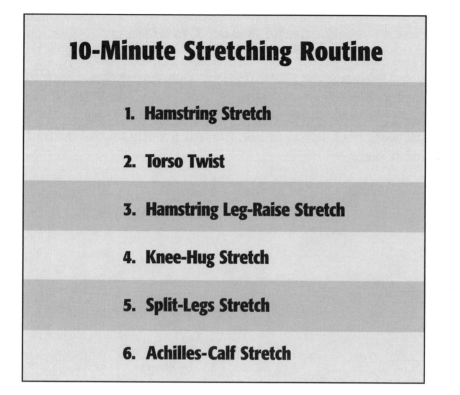

10-Minute Stretching Routine

1. **Hamstring Stretch**

2. **Torso Twist**

3. **Hamstring Leg-Raise Stretch**

4. **Knee-Hug Stretch**

5. **Split-Legs Stretch**

6. **Achilles-Calf Stretch**

"Ready, Set, GO!" - just do it!

Stretching hurts every time I perform the 10-Minute Stretching Routine. But in every case, when the routine is finished, I feel much better than when I started.

On days when I feel really stiff (in other words, most days), I have a motivational cue that I silently say to myself: "get tough...and get focused," and I move into the (not-so-comfortable) hold position.

When my mind begins to play tricks on me about why I can afford to skip stretching today, I immediately quit thinking, move into the start position, take a deep breath, say to myself silently, *"Ready, Set, GO!"* and pull down to the hold position for 30 seconds. I use the "Ready, Set, GO" self-motivation cue with all forms of training.

Ten minutes of exercise has been shown by researchers to improve mood and vigor and decrease fatigue. (Exercise duration and mood state: how much is enough to feel better? 2001, Hansen).

5. Split-Legs Stretch

There are four parts to this stretching position. Start by sitting on the floor and position your legs as illustrated in the first photo. If you are new to flexibility training, remain in the starting stretch-hold position (slightly leaning toward the foot) for 30 seconds.

Start position

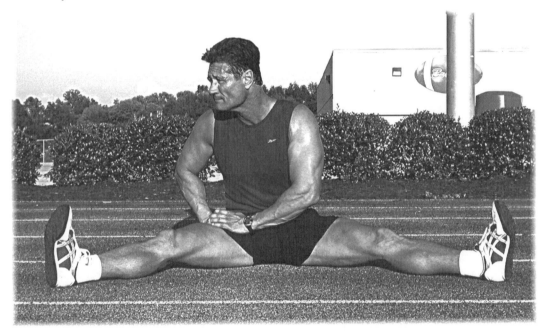

Next, move in slow motion to the "pull right" stretch-hold position. Keep your legs straight, toes up, and very slowly pull your chest toward your right knee. Hold it for 30 seconds. Then pull your chest to the left knee for the 30-second stretch-hold.

Pull right position

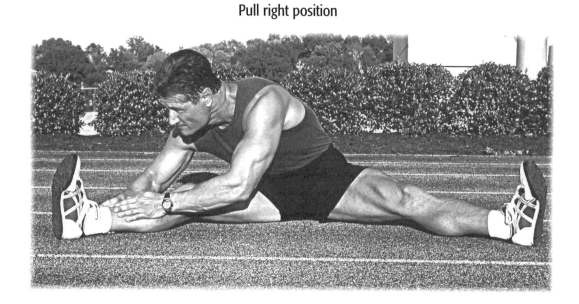

For the final stretching position of this exercise, pull down to the center for 30 seconds in the stretch-hold position shown below.

Center

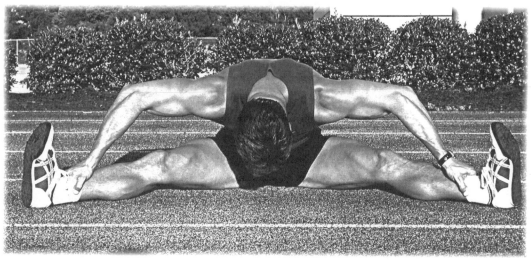

Photographs by Kathy Campbell

6. Achilles - Calf Stretch

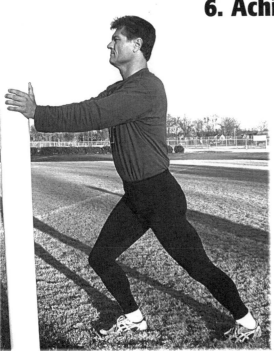

Achilles - Calf Stretch; body straight, forward lean, bent at the ankle, no bouncing, hold for 30 seconds.

Reverse legs and fully stretch Achilles and Calf

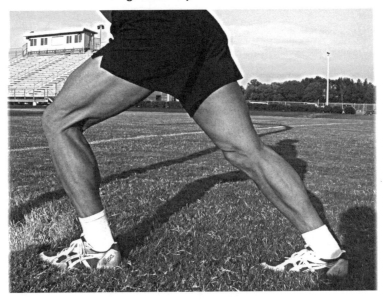

Optional Stretching Positions
Hamstring Stretching

Physicians are called on to think about exercise for the aging population as a "medical prescription" that should include training for flexibility, strength, and endurance. (Aging and Physical Activity, 2000, Leach).

Hamstrings, calves, ankles, and the lower back benefit from the following stretching positions. In the bent, split-legs stretching position demonstrated by personal trainer Bambi LaFont, RN, (age 44, and mother of two) slightly turn toes inward to stretch the outer calves and ankles. This exercise can substitute for the #5. Split-Legs Stretch.

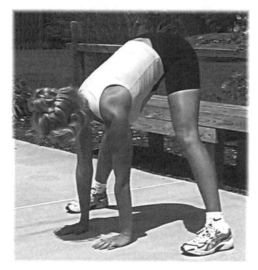

Slightly press down on
thigh to stretch hamstring

The hamstring stretching exercise shown on the right may substitute for the #1 Hamstring Stretch.

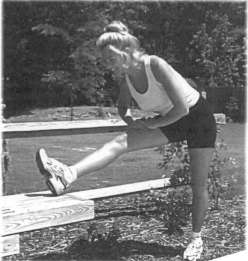

Side Torso Stretch

This stretching position targets the upper body, trunk, abs, ribcage and upper back. Move into this position and hold for 30 seconds on both sides as shown by Kristi McCarver, Shay Ingram (below) and Dr. Cristi Doll (left), author of *The 10 Foods That Should Never Touch a Woman's Lips.*

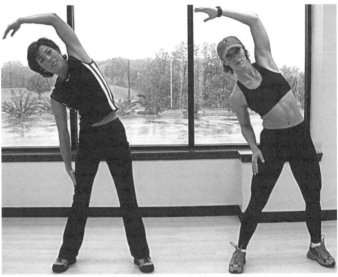

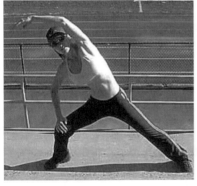

Butterfly Stretch

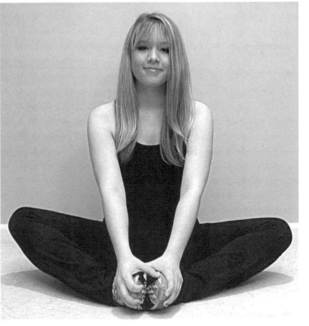

Lower-Back Stretch

The basic Lower-Back Stretch is performed by personal trainer, Melanie Buchholz, JD, (age 40, mother of three). Lying facedown, place hands under shoulders to start. Slowly press upward. As you "feel the limit" in your lower back, stop and hold for 30 seconds. Yoga practitioners call this the "Cobra" pose.

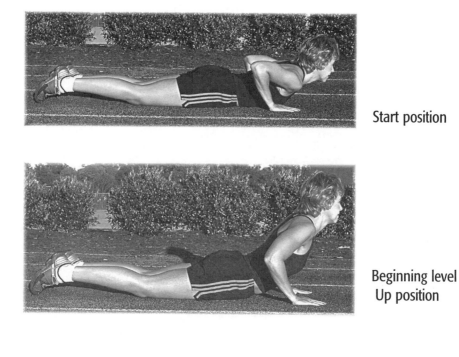

Start position

Beginning level
Up position

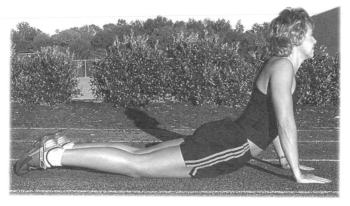

Advanced
Up position

Stretching for Children

Research shows that stretching can prevent injury in children. Researchers conclude that there is a strong association between decreased flexibility and ankle injury in children (*Limited dorsiflexion predisposes to injuries of the ankle in children*, 2000, Tabritzi). Children can easily perform the 10-Minute Stretching Routine.

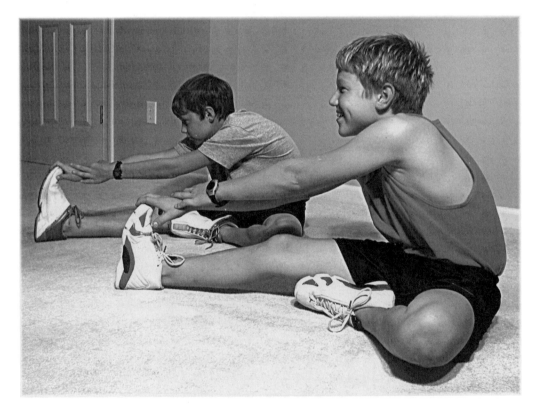

John Campbell and Scott Metcalf demonstrate the
first stretching position of 10-Minute Stretching Routine

Upper-Body Flexibility

Upper-body stretching may be performed with the 10-Minute Stretching Routine, independently, or the *Ready, Set, GO! Fitness* way and save time by multi-tasking upper body flexibility training with resistance training.

During the 1-minute recovery between weightlifting sets, simply take 30 seconds to stretch one side of the upper body. Repeat for the other side during a following set.

NOTE: Upper-Body Flexibility Training

To save time, multi-task exercises by stretching the bodypart being worked between sets during strength training

---

Stretch the body part being worked - is a good rule to follow during weight training. Just like in the 10-Minute Stretching Routine, slowly move to the "fully stretched position" and hold for 30 seconds. In order to maximize results and reduce risk of injury, do not bounce during stretching. Once in the fully stretched position, "feel the limit" and the slight discomfort (at the limit), hold for 30 seconds, and slowly ease out of the position.

Even at advanced levels of fitness, adding stretching to weight training can cause initial soreness, and even injury. As with any new exercise addition, gradually add "flexibility fundamentals" into your resistance training. Remember, no fast movements and move in slow motion as you move into and out of stretching positions.

The following photographs show methods of stretching the major upper body muscle groups - chest, shoulders, and upper back.

Using the rest periods between sets to stretch the working muscle group produces strength gain. *"Data revealed a 16.5 lb. strength gain for the strength training only group while the stretching group had a 19.6 lb. increase, an almost 20 percent greater strength gain,"* 2001, Wayne Westcott, Ph.D., Senior Fitness Director, South Shore YMCA , Quincy, MA.

Upper-Back Stretch

The Hammer Throw Stretch resembles the Olympic event. Grab a stationary bar as illustrated. Lean backward to fully stretch the upper-back muscles (lats). Then lean slightly to the left (fully stretching the left lat muscle), and hold 30 seconds. Repeat, leaning to the right. Perform this while working your upper back during strength training.

Hammer Throw Stretch

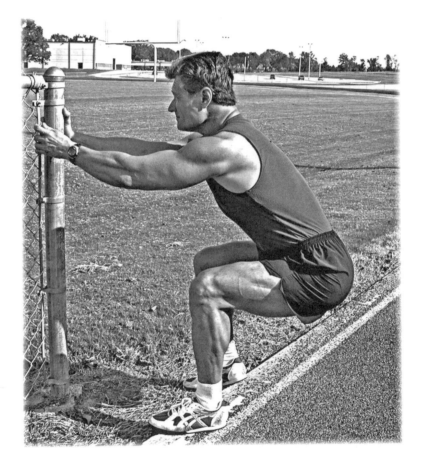

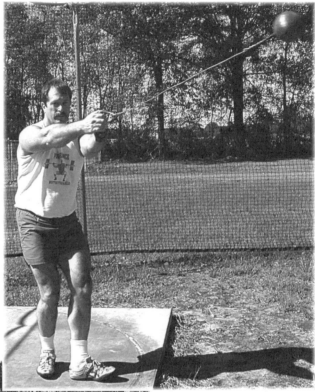

The Hammer Throw Stretch resembles the actual Olympic event. Orthopedic surgeon, Dr. Larry Schrader, All American, masters track and field hammer thrower, uses the Sprint 8 and strength training for general conditioning and preparation for masters track and field competitions

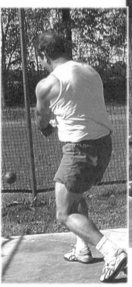

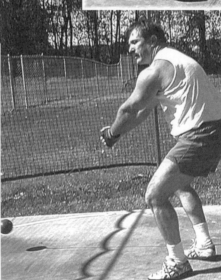

Chest Stretch

The Javelin Throw Stretch shown in the illustration is very effective in stretching the chest muscles. This stretching position is similar to the position you assume before throwing a javelin — palm up, extended arm.

Use the Javelin Throw Stretch while working your chest. Keep the arm stationary and extended, *palm up,* back straight, and chest out. Once in this position, lean forward and "feel the limit" in your chest. Hold for 30 seconds. Repeat on the other side.

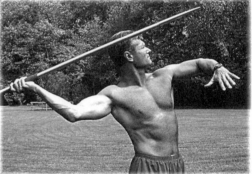

Javelin Throw Stretch

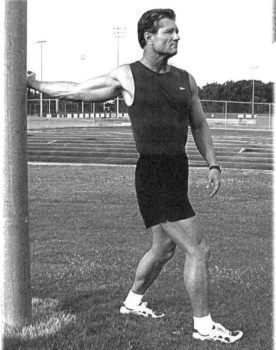

Keeping your palm up (just like throwing the javelin) moves the target area to the chest.

Shoulder Stretch

The Discus Throw Stretch resembles the shoulder movement of throwing a discus. Hold a stationary bar *(palm down)*, with your body upright and chest out, lean forward, and fully stretch the shoulder. Hold for 30 seconds.

Repeat on the other side. Perform this stretch when working shoulders.

Discus Throw Stretch

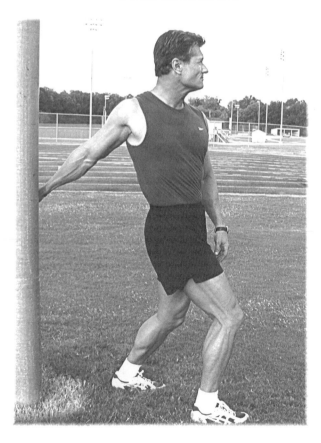

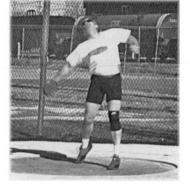

Frank Broadus, Masters Track and Field champion discus thrower and shot-putter from Louisville, KY.

Conclusion

Stretching is a major component of a total fitness plan. It has numerous health benefits in addition to the muscle, joint and ligament benefits of increasing flexibility.

The 10-Minute Stretching Routine is designed for all ages and fitness levels. This routine is programmed into all of the Fitness Plans in Chapter 11.

Keep your book open and you'll memorize the 10-Minute Stretching Routine in just a few sessions. The stretching will make you feel great (once you're finished), and it will help tone your muscles in just the right places.

Remember, flexibility training is unlike other forms of fitness training where you typically experience quick results. It may take several weeks before you see improvement. Hang in there; positive results will come with persistence.

Truthfully, stretching can be somewhat painful initially (especially if you're naturally tight like me), so when your mind starts playing games about passing on the stretching routine, just say to yourself, "Ready, Set, GO!" and start the routine.

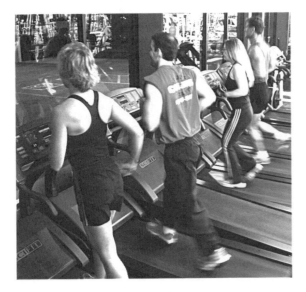

Experienced endurance athletes know, especially long-distance runners, that endurance-trained athletes have greater muscle tightness than most people and need extra flexibility training, (*Lower extremity muscular flexibility in long distance runners*, 1993, Wang).

The next chapter discusses endurance training.

7

Energizing Endurance

Cardio workouts build the endurance base, and this is the foundation for all areas of fitness training discussed in this book. A major new study shows the fastest way to build endurance. And this method is probably much different from what you're thinking, if you're thinking about doing hours of long, slow cardio.

In a major new study by one of the most respected research teams in the world, led by Dr. Martin Gibala, researchers demonstrated that recreationally active adults can actually **double endurance capacity in only two weeks** with a workout almost identical to the 20-minute *Sprint 8* program described in the following chapter. The research summary posted on the National Institutes of Health Website states:

> *We conclude that short sprint interval training (approximately 15 minutes of intense exercise over 2 weeks) increased muscle oxidative potential and* **doubled endurance capacity** *during intense aerobic cycling in recreationally active individuals.*
> (*Six sessions of sprint interval training increases muscle oxidative potential and cycle endurance capacity in humans. 2005, J Appl Physiol. 2005 Jun., Burgomaster KA,*

The importance of this landmark study was published in the *Journal of Applied Physiology* by Dr. Edward Coyle, Director of the prestigious Human Performance Laboratory at the University of Texas in Austin.

Aerobic processes contribute up to 40 percent of the energy used during the first 30 seconds of high-intensity exercise.
(Relative importance of aerobic an anaerobic energy release during short-lasting exhausting bicycle exercise, 1989, Medbo).

Dr. Coyle, who is known for his work with Tour de France champion Lance Armstrong, writes:

This is the first report that you can show large increases in muscle endurance within just two weeks. In today's society, people spend so much time in front of the TV or video screen. It is rare we exercise either intensely or for very long times. Since some people are devoting so little time to exercise, this reminds us how effective or efficient even short amounts of exercise are if performed very intensely.

If you read the first edition of this book in 2000, you learned that exercise-induced HGH can do wonderful things for your body. Now there is conclusive research showing that this type program can significantly improve performance.

Conclusion; long slow cardio is a great starting place to begin building an aerobic base, but this form of training needs to serve as a stepping stone to higher, more productive levels of intensity.

Cardio Training

The goal for cardio training is to achieve the aerobic target heart rate (this changes with age) and maintain that rate for 20 to 30 minutes. Cardio workouts can be performed in many different ways and in many different settings.

Cardio can be performed indoors in aerobic classes at the gym, or on a gym stepper, cycle, rowing machine, elliptical trainer or on a treadmill. And cardio can be performed outside running, cycling, power walking, hiking, swimming and Cross-Country Skiing.

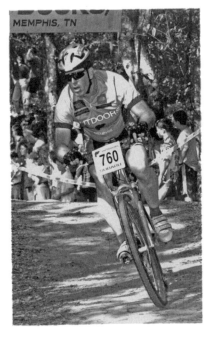

Tom Gee, 55, five-time medalist in the US Cycling, national Masters Championships, qualified for two Olympic Trials and won over 100 State Championship medals.

Figuring Your Target Heart Rate

The typical formula used to calculate aerobic target heart rate is 220 – your age = maximum heart rate. The target range becomes the maximum heart rate x 65 to 85 percent for fit adults.

For beginners, the rate should begin at the 50 percent point and slowly build to 70 percent. The 50 percent target can be easily achieved through power walking (fast walking).

The aerobic target heart rate calculation for age 50:

220 – 50 = 170 max heart rate (HR)

170 x .65 = 110 lower aerobic HR

170 x .85 = 145 highest HR

The aerobic target heart rate range for a 50-year old is between 110 and 145 with the average being 127 heartbeats per minute. During cardio workouts, the goal is to maintain an exercising heart rate of 127 and sustain it for a 20- to 30-minute session. This is a great way to burn calories and build an aerobic base for high-intensity, growth-hormone releasing exercise.

Researchers report that six weeks of amino-acid supplements increased endurance for women untrained in aerobics and weight training. (Effects of exercise training and amino-acid supplementation on body composition and physical performance in untrained women, 2001, Antonio).

An excellent resource for heart health is the book *The Healthy Heart Miracle*, and the Email newsletter produced by Dr. Gabe and Diana Mirkin. This book and newsletter receive my highest recommendation -www.drmirkin.com.

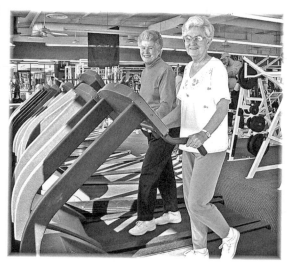

Wilma Diffee & Joan Vidrine
Power Walking on treadmills

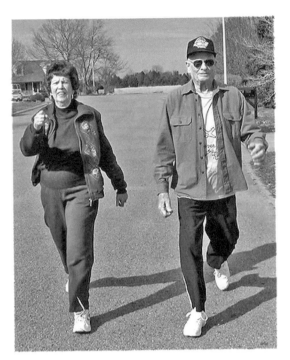

Make Cardio Fun

Bertha Campbell McClenny, 80, my mom, and my step-dad Jacob McClenny, Lt. Col., Air Force (Retired), 87, multi-tasking cardio and the Ready, Set, GO! Sprint 8 by power walking 8 mailboxes in front of their home. Finding a training partner can help motivation if you agree to encourage each other.

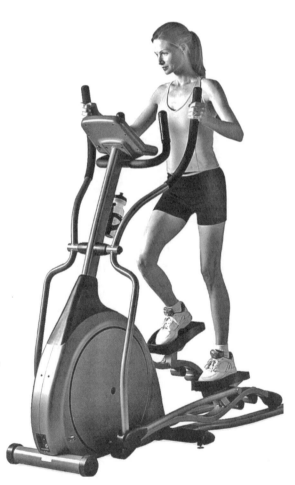

For motivation to continue, it's important to make cardio fun. And there are many ways to do this. Finding an encouraging training partner is helpful. Getting outside is positive, but it's important to plan ahead for bad weather days. Getting high-quality cardio equipment for your home is a great way to fulfill your "Fitness for a Lifetime" commitment.

The award-winning Elliptical Trainer shown is made by Vision Fitness and it features the *Sprint 8* described in the following chapter.

For retail stores and locations offering home cardio equipment with the *Sprint 8* program visit www.visionfitness.com and click "retailer locator."

Aerobic vs. Anaerobic Training

The debate of aerobic exercise verses anaerobic training is shortsighted and misses the theme of this book. It is not a question of one over the other. These two forms of training are interrelated and are both vital components of a comprehensive fitness plan.

The endurance base - built by aerobic exercise - makes anaerobic exercise possible.

Does cardio training increase HGH? It's possible, but it may take two training sessions during the same day. If you are *not* a time-crunched adult and have plenty of time, you can certainly try this.

Researchers show that a second endurance training session during the same day will increase HGH (*Increased neuroendocrine response to a repeated bout of endurance exercise*, 2001, Ronsen).

Researchers show that the health profile and total body fitness for women can be improved dramatically with aerobics and resistance training. (Resistance training combined with bench-step aerobics enhances women's health profile, 2001, Kraemer).

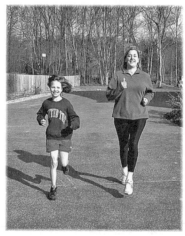

Cindy and Halie Miller, mother and daughter, doing the Sprint 8 Workout in their driveway.

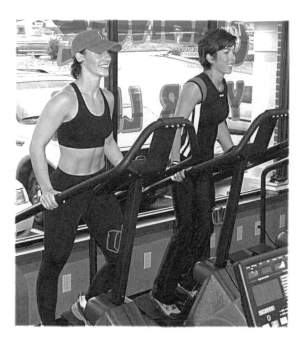

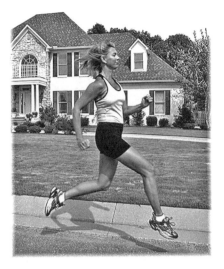

Time Crunched?
Multi-Task Aerobic Training with Anaerobic Training

Accomplishing both aerobic and anaerobic training simultaneously may be achieved by multi-tasking exercises in your fitness plan. Sprinting, bleacher running, and plyometric drills achieve anaerobic training levels. And using a brief, 1.5-minute recovery between sprints will keep the heart rate over cardio target heart rate during the workout. The Sprint 8 does this.

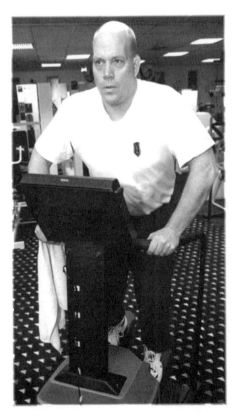

Educator Rick Wolf Sets the Example

Educator Rick Wolf typically runs outside - even when it's 20 below - but he uses a cardio stepper unit on rainy days.

He writes about the exhilarating experience of performing anaerobic exercise before beginning the school day:

It's just after 6:00 AM and I've just finished my first of five "Sprint 8's" that will be a part of this morning's run. Never mind that it's 5 below zero. I'm 53 years old now, I'm feeling better than ever and it's going to be a beautiful dawn. I can accomplish anything today!
- Rick Wolf, Reading, PA

Interval Training

Interval training programs are designed to reduce running time per mile and increase endurance. It's possible for triathletes, marathon, and mid-distance runners to reduce their running times significantly with interval training and sprinting. Researchers conclude:

> *The results indicate that anaerobic power is significantly related to distance running performance and may explain a meaningful percentage of variability in 10-km run time. Therefore, it may be beneficial for distance runners to* **supplement aerobic training with some power and speed development such as plyometrics and sprinting.** (The relationship between field tests of anaerobic power and 10-km run performance, 2001, J Strength Cond Res, Sinnett AM).

Interval training is discussed more in the next chapter *The Sprint 8 - Targeting Exercise-Induced HGH.*

Research demonstrates "significant differences" in the release of human growth hormone by anaerobic and aerobic exercise. Anaerobic training clearly achieves HGH release. (Effect of anaerobic and aerobic exercise of equal duration and work on plasma growth hormone levels, 1984, Vanhelder).

Dr. Mike Trexler, 52, USA Track & Field masters sprint champion, uses the Sprint 8 Workout with interval training to increase speed and endurance. Dr. Trexler has appeared as a fitness expert on national TV programs with Katie Couric, Bryant Gumbel, and Leeza Gibbons

Bleacher Running Multi-Tasks
Anaerobic and Aerobic Exercise

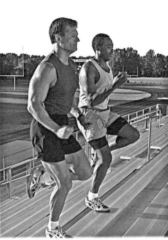

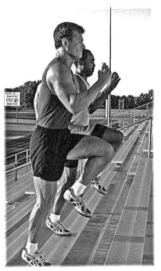

Photographs by Kathy Campbell

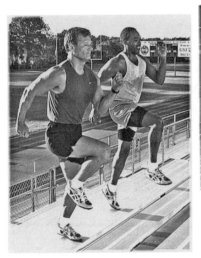

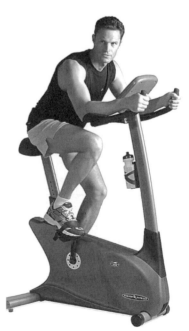

Running bleachers with my running partner, Nate Robertson, State Games 100 and 200-meter sprint champion

Whether running sprints on bleachers on a nice day, or pushing the Sprint 8 button on an upright bike at home when it's cold outside, anaerobic and aerobic exercise can be performed together for powerful results

Impact of Anaerobic Exercise on Heart Rate

The following graph illustrates the impact of the Sprint 8 on heart rate. During the sprint, the heart rate rises far above the aerobic target heart rate after the first few sprints. It continues to remain above the target heart rate during the 1.5 to 2-minute walk-back to the starting line recovery.

Target Heart Rate During Sprint 8 Workout

Performance of multi-tasking the anaerobic Sprint 8 Workout and aerobic exercise measured by heart rate for 20 minutes

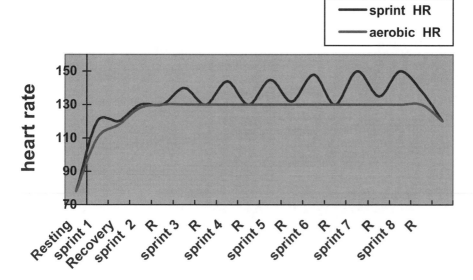

Sprint 8 Workout with 1.5 - 2 minute recovery during walk-back to start, compared to aerobic target heart rate

Road Running?
Change Your Shoes Frequently

Long distance runners need to replace running shoes much more frequently than you may expect. Mileage, body weight, and running surfaces cause wear on running shoes. Typically, every three months (and less for some runners), it's time to get new shoes. Street running requires shoes with maximum padding.

Don't be stingy on running shoes. Running is not an expensive sport. So what if you spend 25 cents a mile on shoes if it prevents permanent damage to your knees, hips, and lower back? You may save thousands of dollars in future healthcare bills. Changing shoes frequently may help to reduce stress fractures that are sometimes caused by street running. This can become a significant problem for long distance runners (*Interventions for preventing and treating stress fractures and stress reactions of bones of the lower limbs in young adults*, 2000, Gillespie).

Researchers show that absorbing insoles can reduce the risk of stress fractures, and additional calcium nutrition may be helpful.

Springbak makes "Performance-Boosting Speedsoles" for athletes involved in running sports. These insoles are very thin, light, and provide solid shock absorption; www.springbak.com. Because these insoles are thin, they fit in dress shoes and are great when standing on hard floors.

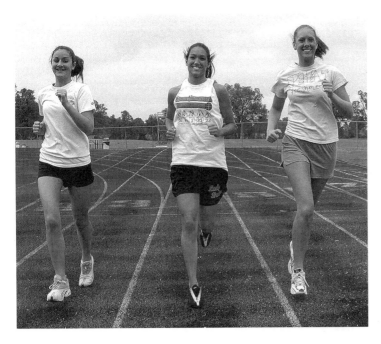

Carrie Beth Henson, Christine Campbell, and Kacie Fite running on the track in off-season training

Bone & Joint Smart Training

It's not only bone & joint smart to back off the hard surface mileage a few days a week, the Gibala endurance study shows that sprint training three days a week can double endurance in as little as two weeks.

With this statement, let me quickly add that if you are a long distance runner and you want to improve performance, your training needs to replicate the actual movement of your sport, long distance running. And you must perform long distance, race pace (and faster) training - just not everyday.

The endurance athletes that I've worked with seem to get best results with one long run a week at race pace, one mid-distance run at faster than race pace with the Sprint 8 to finish the workout, and two speed training days.

Speed training consists of the Sprint 8 on both days, and on one of the days, follow the Sprint 8 with 4 x 150 meter sprints.

Protect your knees. The risk of knee arthritis is eight times greater in individuals with a previous knee injury. (A case-control study to investigate the relationship between the low and moderate levels of physical activity and osteoarthritis of the knee using data collected as part of the Allied Dunbar National Fitness Survey, 2001, Sutton).

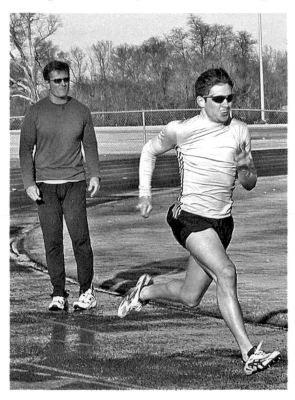

John Fischer, sub 4.30 miler and age group, nationally ranked high school triathlete running 4 X 150s during speed training

Conclusion

The "missing ingredient" in most fitness plans today is anaerobic training that includes a slow, methodical, and progressive build-up period in concert with a knowledgable primary physician as a partner in the process. You must have an aerobic base to build on before you step up to anaerobic training.

The Fitness Plans in Chapter 11 contain workouts called "Cardio-20" and "Cardio-30" (this means 20 or 30 minutes) of long, slow aerobic training. However, when you're ready, consider stepping-up your intensity during all of your cardio workouts by multi-tasking anaerobic and aerobic training. You'll discover exactly how to do this in the following chapter.

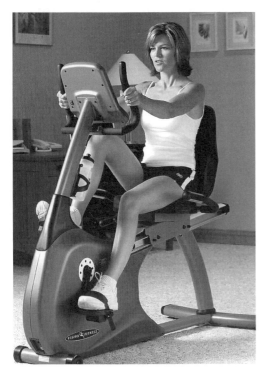

The award-winning Vision Fitness Recumbent Bike features the *Sprint 8* program described in Chapter 8.

Simply press the *"Sprint 8"* button and you're on your way to a great 20-minute anaerobic/ aerobic workout.

Sprint 8 is designed to make the body produce the most powerful body fat cutting, muscle toning, energy improving substance known to science.

For more information about Vision Fitness home cardio equipment, see www.visionfitness.com for details

8

Sprint 8

Targeting Exercise-Induced Growth Hormone

Anaerobic workouts improve performance for athletes of all ages. And anaerobic training accelerates the release of exercise-induced growth hormone like no other form of exercise. Yet, this aspect of training is often missing in fitness plans today.

Dr. Declan Connolly, Director of the Human Performance Lab at the University of Vermont says, "Loss of **strength and speed** is potentially of greater concern in the aging population than loss of cardiovascular fitness. Appropriate resistance and anaerobic training can help ensure good muscle strength and function into older age."

To successfully **add anaerobic training** to your fitness program, you will need to strengthen your fast and super-fast muscle fiber. Your exercise selection needs to be comprehensive and include exercises that develop your slow-twitch (type I), fast-twitch (IIa), and super-fast (IIx) fiber - slowly and incrementally.

Spending several weeks babying your hamstrings, calves, quads and Achilles by progressively building your fast muscle fiber, is a wise strategy. The fast-muscle fiber will become strong as it adapts to speed training and explosive lifting, if you'll take a methodical, progressive approach.

We conclude that short sprint interval training (approximately 15 minutes of intense exercise over 2 weeks) increased muscle oxidative potential and doubled endurance capacity during intense aerobic cycling in recreationally active individuals. (Six sessions of sprint interval training increases muscle oxidative potential and cycle endurance capacity in humans), 2005, J Appl Physiol. Jun., Burgomaster KA,

Sprint 8 Can be Performed
Many Different Ways!

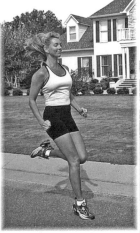
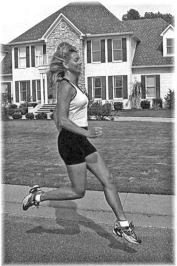
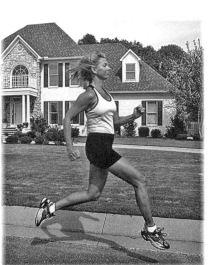

Personal Trainer, Bambi LaFont, BS, RN, age 44, performs the Sprint 8 Workout at home

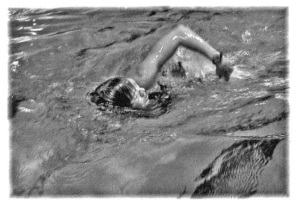

Sprint swimming

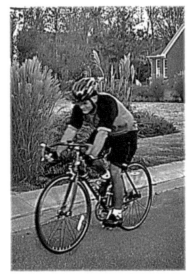

U.S. Masters Swimming www.usms.org is an excellent resource

Chris LaFont sprint cycling

Sprint-trained athletes can increase HGH levels to 10 times the normal level, report researchers at Loughborough University, England. And sprint training can produce 82% more exercise-induced HGH than endurance training.

This is due to *"peak power output and peak blood lactate response to the sprint."* In fitness training, only an intense, anaerobic workout can produce a significant increase in growth hormone. (*Growth hormone responses to treadmill sprinting in sprint- and endurance-trained athletes*, 1996, Nevill).

Whether you run, cycle, or swim the Sprint 8, or choose another method, anaerobic training is absolutely necessary in a comprehensive fitness plan.

Now I wish I could tell you the Sprint 8 only takes 20 minutes, will get you in great physical condition, and it's easy. I can't.

However, I *can* tell you that the Sprint 8 will get you in great physical condition, it only takes 20 minutes, and it can cover a few not-so-healthy meals.

But this workout is intense. You'll find, however, that the benefits far outweigh the effort. And in just 20 minutes, you will have finished an incredible workout.

Comparing the ability of different types of exercise to produce human growth hormone release, anaerobic training receives the highest marks from medical researchers. (Hormonal and metabolic response to three types of exercise of equal duration and external work output, 1985, Vanhelder).

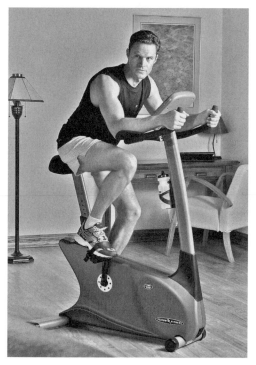

Does The Sprint 8 Workout Work?

Letter from Harvey Fischer

I was getting ready to turn 50, and I was not in good shape. I didn't have energy to exercise.

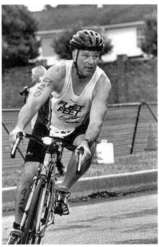

I felt bad, and I was overweight. I tried numerous fitness programs that were big on promises, but none worked.

*Then I read **Ready, Set, Go! Synergy Fitness** by Phil Campbell, and it made sense, and I knew this program would get results.*

I made the Eight Week Commitment, exactly one year ago. For the Sprint 8 Workout, I could only walk initially and did the weight training at the local YMCA.

***ONE YEAR LATER** - I feel better at 51 than I did at 31. My progress with the Ready, Set, GO! plan has been beyond my wildest imagination! Not only have I lost weight, I have been able to enter several masters competitions that you recommend.*

I've completed six 5K runs, five triathlons. I finished 1st in my age group in the one mile run and 2nd in the 800 in a Masters Track & Field event.

Ready, Set, Go! has been my guide to better health and it has helped me to become an athlete again. The Sprint 8 Workout and interval training workouts in the book have not only helped in running, but in the other areas as well. I do the Sprint 8 with swimming and biking and it has been the biggest factor improving my triathlon times. My PR (Personal Record) for the sprint is 1:09 at a Triathlon. My next goal is to compete with my son John, age 16, in a Half Ironman in May.

Thank you for putting all the information in one book. Most of all, thank you for helping me get my health back. I recommend this book to everyone.

Sincerely,

Harvey Fischer, triathlete

Don't Let the Word *Sprint* Frighten You!

The Sprint 8 doesn't necessarily mean running full speed. It doesn't even mean running. There are many ways to perform the Sprint 8. If you are age 70, you'll need eight repetitions of some type of anaerobic exercise lasting 10 to 30 seconds, with 1.5 to 2 minutes of recovery in between. A home recumbent bike or power walking would be a good place to start.

If you are age 17 and in shape, an athlete, or middle-aged and fit, then the intensity of your Sprint 8 will need to be at a higher level to achieve HGH release benchmarks.

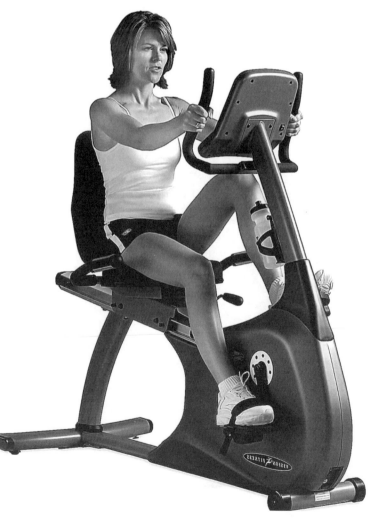

The Sprint 8 only takes 20 minutes and it's a powerful tool in any fitness plan. In fact, researchers suggest that 20 minutes of exercise at 90 percent intensity may even be a suitable method for testing deficiencies of growth hormone secretion, (Sutton, 1976).

With the correct levels of intensity, great workouts don't need hours of your time in the gym. The Sprint 8 will get this aspect of fitness training done for you in 20 minutes.

"We conclude that the GH response to acute aerobic exercise is augmented with repeated bouts of exercise. " (1997 Nov, *Human growth hormone response to repeated bouts of aerobic exercise,* J Appl Physiol, Kanaley JA).

Sprint 30 Seconds or LESS Rule

The running version of the Sprint 8 will reach all HGH-release benchmarks quickly because running sprints is higher in intensity than most other forms of sprinting.

When running sprints, you are carrying your full body weight. When swimming sprints, the water is supporting some of your body weight, and when cycling sprints, the bike is supporting a significant amount of your body weight. And your muscles don't have to work as hard when your body weight is supported.

This means that you can run a sprint and cover 60 meters in 8 to 12 seconds, or pedal hard and fast to sprint on a recumbent cycle for 30 seconds and achieve a similar level of exercise intensity.

Important point, whatever method of sprinting you choose, make sure that you cannot go for much more than 30 seconds. If you're sprinting on a cardio unit that's not programmed with the Sprint 8, and stop the sprint at 30 seconds when you could have gone for 45 seconds, this is a mistake. The intensity is not great enough.

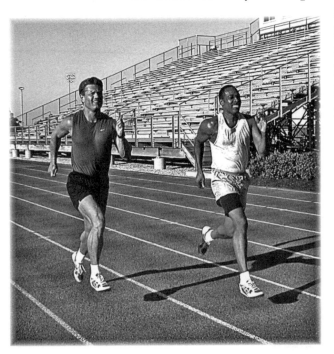

Running warm-up sprints with my main running partner, Nate Robertson

To get the full impact of Sprint 8, you'll need to pedal at an intensity level that gets you really winded and wanting to stop around 10 to 15 seconds. But hang on for 30 seconds when sprinting on cardio equipment.

We're talking about real intensity. Now, if you are a 400-meter sprinter trained to handle lactate for 45 seconds, perhaps you can use a longer time for the sprint. Maybe. After training thousands of athletes to run faster during Speed Camps, my experience is that anyone, endurance athletes included, will subconsciously pace when the sprint is over 30 seconds. And pacing is the enemy of intensity!

When running the Sprint 8, you don't need a track although a track is more comfortable and typically safer than the streets. All you need is a straightway approximately 60 meters (70 yards) long and around 10 meters to slow-down.

After warm-up, the first sprint should begin at a jogging pace (approximately 30 percent speed/intensity) and progressively build to 50 percent speed/intensity.

After passing the finish mark (mailbox, yard line, tree), gradually slow down to avoid injury. To avoid common "stop/start" hamstring injuries, take a full 10 yards to slow-down and stop after the sprint.

The gradual slow-down at the end of the sprint is extremely important because injuries occur most frequently during starting and stopping. Ease into the start, and ease off the sprint after crossing the finish line.

"Although walking is popular, few people do enough walking to benefit their health. Those who walk as well as engage in other physical activities appear more likely to achieve recommended levels of activity." (Relative influences of individual, social environmental, and physical environmental correlates of walking, Am J Public Health. 2003, Giles-Corti B).

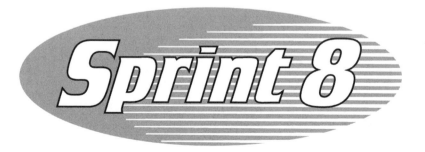

Do not allow the quest for the endurance aspect of "speed endurance" to overshadow the speed work. To build speed, take the full recovery (during the walk-back between sprints) so you have adequate energy for speed technique improvement and power development during training.

Make sure and take the full 1.5 to 2-minute recovery by walking back (at a casual pace) to the starting line. The walking recovery will enable you to put more intensity into the following sprint.

The second sprint repetition will begin at a 40 percent pace and progressively increase intensity to 60 percent speed/intensity. Likewise, the third sprint starts at a 50 percent pace and builds to 70 percent intensity. The progressive, build-up sprint program is outlined in the chart on page 158.

First Time Running Sprints

On the first day, even if you are fit and can run a marathon, at the most, only perform four sprints unless you are sprint-conditioned. And slowly add one or two sprints to your workout every session until you get to the full eight sprints.

Once you are sprint-conditioned, the last three to four sprints should be at 80 percent plus intensity level and even up to 90 to 95 percent speed/intensity - once your body can handle this level of intensity.

When you're sweating, out-of-breath, and your muscles are slightly burning, you'll know you have reached the HGH-release benchmarks.

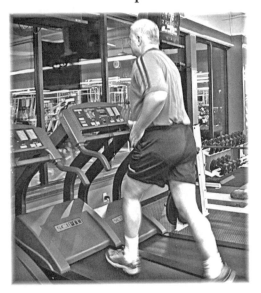

Dr. Randall Bush runs the Sprint 8 on a treadmill by increasing the elevation & speed during the 8 sprints, and decreasing elevation and speed during the 90-second recovery periods

WARNING!
Sprinting & heat can be dangerous!

Since 1953, over 100 U.S. football athletes have died on the field. An expert who appeared on the television show *Real Sports* to discuss the deaths of two athletes - a pro-football player who died during summer camp, and the death of a 5'10" - 280 pound high school football player who died while practicing in the hot sun for six hours - provided insightful information about what happened. The deaths, he said, were caused by "**a malfunction of the heat regulation system in the brain.**"

The combination of extreme heat, heavy clothing, lack of fluids, and sprint-type anaerobic sports like football, can become very dangerous. Common sense with anaerobic training is a must! Remember, when in doubt about any aspect of fitness training, contact your physician for clearance.

Drink Water!

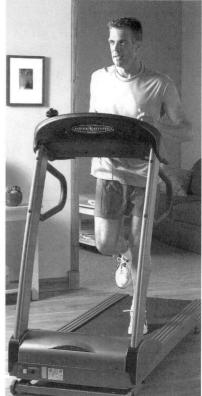

If you are running sprints outdoors, it's not a bad idea to drink a sip of water between every sprint. I do this.

Anaerobic training is demanding, and it increases body temperature very quickly. Not only is hydration a safety issue, but researchers show that exercise-induced HGH will be significantly decreased when you don't get enough fluids during exercise, (Peyreign, 2001).

On days when the temperature isn't cooperating with your training schedule, indoor training is a wise strategy.

The Sprint 8 is featured on new Vision Fitness home treadmills (shown right). This is a beefed-up treadmill to handle the demands of high-intensity

TRAINING TIP
Expect it to be difficult to perform anaerobic training some days. On the days when I do not feel like training, simply saying "Ready, Set, GO," to myself (silently) is my personal cue to "get tough" on myself, get focused, start, and finish the workout.

The following chart shows sprint intensity for running the Sprint 8 once you've spent eight weeks progressively building the fast-twitch fiber and aerobic base to accommodate this high level of intensity. Again, make sure you have your physician's approval before starting an anaerobic exercise program, drink plenty of fluids during the workout, and resist the temptation to run too fast too soon.

Sprint 8 Workout
Progressive Anaerobic Running Sprints

1st Sprint	Begin jogging; build to **50 percent** speed/intensity. Walk-back recovery (1.5 to 2 minutes)
2nd Sprint	Begin 40% pace, build to **60%**
3rd Sprint	Begin 50%, build to **70%**
4th Sprint	Begin 60%, build to **80%**
5th Sprint	Begin 70%, build to **90%**
6th Sprint	Build to **95%**
7th Sprint	95%
8th Sprint	95%
Cool-down	Walk or jog 2 minutes

Attention Ex-Jocks - Warning!

Many former athletes implementing the Sprint 8 Workout begin feeling so good during the first two to three weeks that they decide to see just how fast they can run during the last sprint.

Pulled hamstrings are the results of not slowly and progressively rebuilding the fast-twitch fibers for 6 to 8 weeks. Slow-twitch muscles have been maintained through the years and feel good, but without realizing it, fast-twitch muscles have atrophied and decreased in strength, size, and flexibility.

Don't be misled by the feeling of your strong slow-twitch muscles; it will take several months of rebuilding the fast-twitch muscles before you can push the intensity levels beyond 70 percent speed.

Whether you are 17 or 70, exercise intensity is relative to age and conditioning. Your anaerobic program should be fun, fast, and effective - at any age. However, keep in mind that the Sprint 8 is very demanding and could be hazardous to your health.

A slow, build-up period and a physical exam by your physician, are necessary before performing high-intensity exercise. Start with two to four progressive sprints the first day and make them easy. Progressively build by adding one or two sprint repetitions during future workouts. Once you get up to eight sprints, then begin adding speed intensity.

Expect some soreness after the first few Sprint 8 workouts. Even for the young and fit, sprinting works muscles not touched by most exercises. And keep in mind that sprinting requires more warm-up time.

Sprinting on Cardio Equipment

The Sprint 8 is now featured in award-winning Vision Fitness commercial and home cardio equipment.

When I wrote *Ready, Set, Go! Synergy Fitness* in 2000, most cardio equipment companies were looking for ways to make higher quality cardio equipment. Vision Fitness, having already achieved this, had a different goal: to create fitness equipment that would make it easier and more engaging for people to achieve a better, healthier life.

Vision Fitness investigated the new research I cited in my book and invited me to their headquarters for a presentation of my SPRINT 8 program.

Vision Fitness executives didn't just take my word for it.

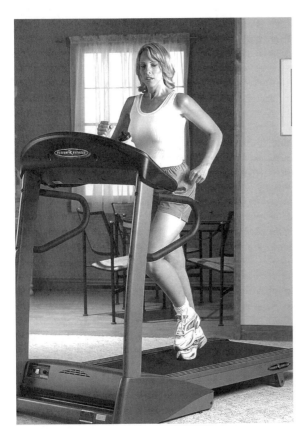

They wanted to test drive the SPRINT 8 workout themselves. Senior managers, product engineers, their wives (this is a family-oriented company), and numerous others in the Vision Fitness family took the Eight Week Challenge in my book. They performed the SPRINT 8 workout three times a week for eight weeks.

The results they achieved in body fat loss, muscle toning, and energy enhancement mirrored what the researchers stated about exercise-induced HGH. *"Exercise-induced growth hormone release mimics taking growth hormone injections,"* which on average case will yield a 14% loss in body fat and an 8% increase in lean muscle mass.

They were so thrilled with the results that they decided to add the SPRINT 8 program to their cardio equipment and share it with their customers.

Visionary Leadership

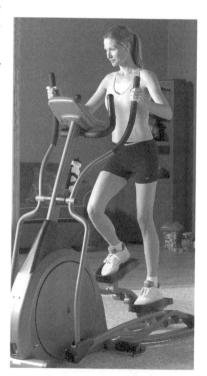

In the first edition of my book, running sprints was the primary method for performing the Sprint 8.

Today, due to the visionary leadership of Nathan Pyles, Greg Waters, Chris Cox and the Vision Fitness team, you can easily perform the Sprint 8 at home on an elliptical trainer, step-thru recumbent bike, upright bike, or on a new Vision Fitness treadmill that's been specially designed to handle the extra load of high-intensity sprinting. Just hop on, touch the Sprint 8 button, and you're on your way to a great 20-minute workout designed to target exercise-induced growth hormone.

For more information, visit a retail fitness store specializing in home fitness equipment and give the Sprint 8 a test drive. There's a list of retail fitness stores offering the Sprint 8 posted at www.visionfitness.com under "Retailer Locator."

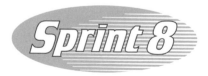

When shopping for home cardio equipment to continue training on bad weather days, save drive time, or train safe in your home, look for this Sprint 8 trademark at your favorite home fitness retail store

How to Improve Athletic Performance

Training intensity, n*ot training volume*, determines performance improvement. A common mistake made by   athletes is thinking "more training is better." It's natural to think this, but over-training can harm your body and slow your progress.

The research is clear, "intensity," and not "training volume" is the key factor in improving performance, *(Effects of training on performance in competitive swimming,* 1995, Mujika).

Investigating methods to improve the performance of athletes who are in a slump, researchers show that over-training may be one of the main reasons for slumps, *(Responses to training in cross-country skiers, 1999,* Gaskill).

It's common sense that practicing technique when tired teaches the body to move with poor technique. By moving away from outdated training routines such as traditional slow-tempo lifting and performing strength training specifically for your sport, it's easier than you may think to improve athletic performance.

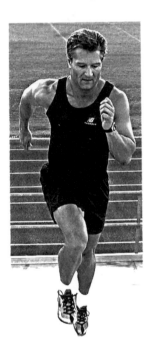

When athletes go to the gym, for example, they usually focus on the traditional exercises that they've read about in magazines, and know how to do. These exercises are great for bodybuilding and developing general strength. But they won't help develop speed unless explosive-lifting techniques are applied to strength training.

Muscles adapt, and lifting with the traditional tempo of up-on-two, down-on-four, will build strong slow-twitch fiber. But it takes strong fast-twitch muscle fiber to score touchdowns, make the tackle, steal second, make the hoop, win the race, or win the gold.

Basically, squatting makes you a better squatter. In test after test, squats do not help vertical jump. Squats build slow muscle fiber, which is positive since that's 40% of your "muscles." Plyometric drills and explosive lifting techniques build the fast (IIa) muscle fiber and the super-fast (IIx) muscle fiber.

Improving Speed

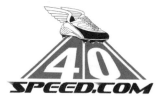

Despite popular belief, running speed is not a genetics-only issue. Genetics has a role, but speed is a skill. And skills can be learned and improved when new techniques are applied.

Clearly, running speed can be improved with correct information, technique coaching, and training. I have several resources I would like to recommend in addition to my speed training Website www.40speed.com.

The book, *Sports Speed,* by Dintiman, Ward and Tellez (Tom Tellez coached Olympian Carl Lewis), is an excellent book specifically aimed at improving all aspects of speed. If you are a high school or college athlete involved in a sport where speed is important, you need the information in this book and the book by Earl Fee. Earl Fee's book, *The Complete Guide to Running,* is an excellent resource - www.feetnessforlife.com.

Perhaps the most informative Website on the Internet concerning sports and coaching is produced by Coach Brian Mackenzie from the UK - www.brianmac.demon.co.uk. It's loaded with reliable information.

MastersTrack.com is an informative Website and *Masters Track & Field News* is packed with great information for masters athletes - www.NationalMastersNews.com. Ross Dunton produces a quality masters track & field Email newsletter - www.coachr.org.

If you're looking for coaching to improve your performance during the college or pro football combines, team training for soccer, baseball, basketball, football, or personal training so you can run your fastest 40 ever, visit www.40speed.com.

Scenes from Speed Camp
www.40speed.com

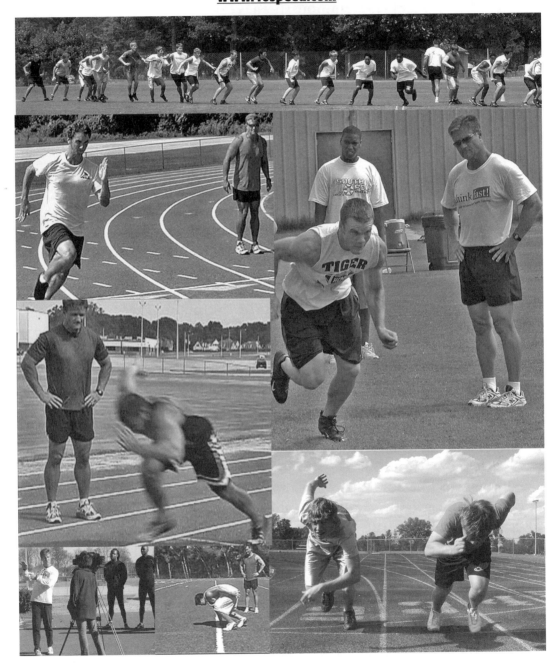

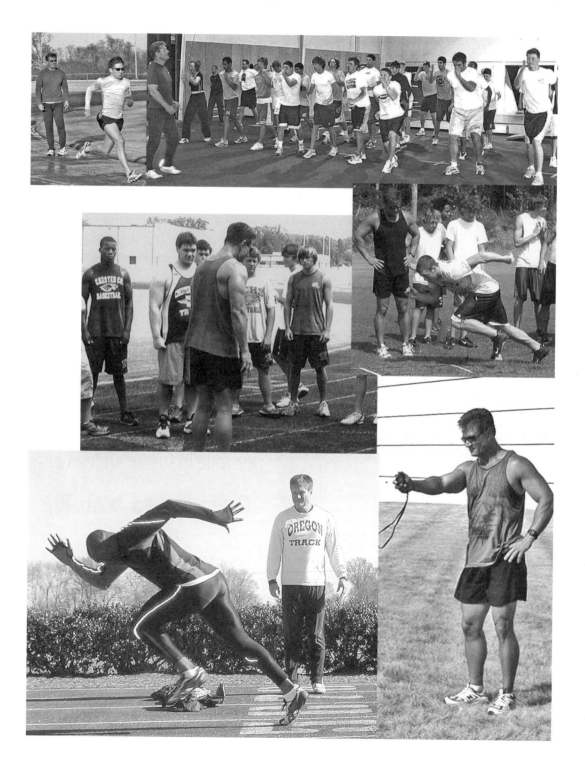

Over-Speed Training

Over-speed training is running at a faster pace than you are capable. The goal is to reprogram the central nervous system and the muscles involved in running to move faster. This is possible with some type of speed-assisted device, running downhill, or running with the wind to your back.

Interval training for marathoners, triathletes, and mid-distance runners is similar to over-speed training for sprinters.

Athletes participating in sports requiring running speed should consider including over-speed training in their training. Elite sprinters looking to shave micro-seconds off their 100-meter and 200-meter times use over-speed training. I've used over-speed training in Speed Camps to help athletes involved in many different sports get faster. And this type of training is very effective.

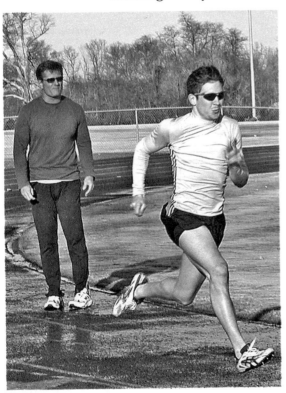

Interval training
improves time
per mile in endurance events

Over-speed training
improves
40 yard dash time
& speed for sports

John Fischer drops his mile time to below 4.30 minutes with speed training

For sprinters, over-speed training can be accomplished by running downhill on a surface with a slight degree slope. Too much slope will hurt, rather than help develop speed technique.

The slope from the center of a football field to the sidelines (drainage slope) is perfect. Also, a 30 foot piece of surgical tubing can be used to pull sprinters for an assisted 10-meter boost.

Over-speed training devices and speed development resources may be purchased at www.power-systems.com.

Interval Training for Distance Runners

Marathon athletes, try this workout to improve your speed and endurance. Add the following interval/sprint over-speed training program two days a week.

Speed Development Workout

- **Warm-up**
- **Sprint 8 Workout**
- **4 reps x 150-meter sprints**
- **10-Minute Stretching Routine**

Remember to walk-back and fully recover during the Sprint 8 and the 150-meter intervals. Resist the temptation to make this an endurance-building workout. Think "speed development and technique" with this workout.

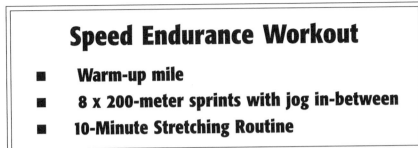

Speed Endurance Workout

- ■ **Warm-up mile**
- ■ **8 x 200-meter sprints with jog in-between**
- ■ **10-Minute Stretching Routine**

Run 200 meters in 28 to 36 seconds, jog at a slow pace the next 200 meters (this completes one lap on a 400-meter track). Sprint the second 200 meters, jog 200 meters. Repeat for four laps total, or eight repetitions of the fast 200s.

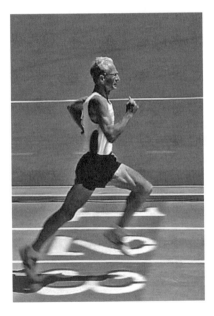

Earl Fee, P.Eng, author of
the highly recommended
The Complete Guide to Running
and masters track & field
champion has set over
30 World Records.
www.feetnessforlife.com

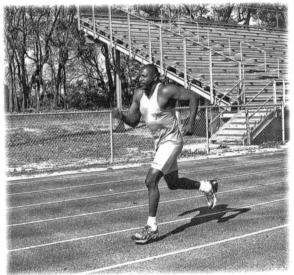

"I feel great when I run sprints. It
keeps the weight off. And I can eat
what I want when I do the Sprint 8."
- Paul Williams, age 43

Secret Weapons
of Speed Development

Developing strong and flexible hip flexors, quads and hamstrings, reducing negative foot speed, and over-speed training are important factors in speed development.

Hip flexors are located at the front top of your thighs and around your hip joints. Hip Flexor Raises (below) target this area. Sit on the edge of the leg-extension machine as shown. Raise the knee as high as possible using the top part of your thigh to perform the work without leaning backward.

Hip Flexor Raises

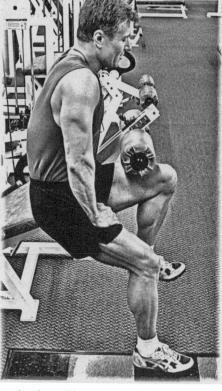

Start

Raised position

Hamstring Development

Your hamstrings should be 75 to 80 percent as strong as your quadriceps (thighs) in a leg extension & leg curl strength test. Experts report that most athletes have hamstrings that are typically only 50 percent as strong as the quads. Chapter 10, Tactical Strength Training, offers a detailed hamstring development program.

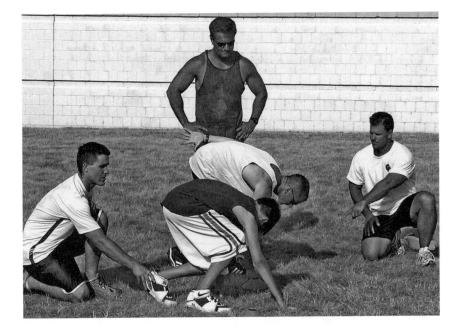

Speed Camp on the Road

Strength training equipment designer for Vision Fitness, Dan Finn and son, Jordan, learning the Combine Start position at Lake Country Athletic Club, Milwaukee, WI. Football coach and head personal trainer, Kris Walter (R) & Travis Bucholtz (L), US Amateur Kick boxing Champion, tweak the starting position

Technique Tip: Run dorsiflexed, land mid-foot, and don't *"reach & pull"* during your stride

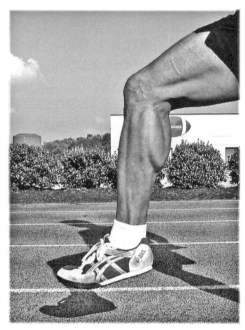

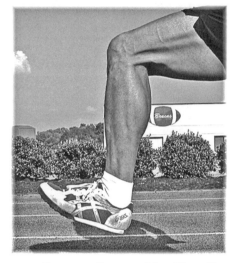

Correct: Foot up "dorsiflexed"

Incorrect:
Foot pointed down

To increase running speed, it's important to strike the surface correctly and eliminate the "reach and pull" motion during the running cycle. Reaching for speed is one of the most common technique mistakes made by runners.

When the foot lands on the surface, the movement shouldn't be a "reach and pull" with the foot. The foot should be dorsiflexed with toes up as shown above and it should strike the surface mid-foot, and land underneath the center of the body.

If your stride is a "reach and pull" movement, you are creating a small braking action with every step. This movement is like driving a car with the parking brake pressed halfway. You can still drive, but it's slow and you're wasting valuable energy.

The lower leg and thigh should be swept backwards at the time of impact, creating an active striking action (backwards). This technique positions the strong "push" muscles of the legs (quads, upper hamstrings, gluts) to move the body forward, rather than using the lower hamstrings to "pull" the body.

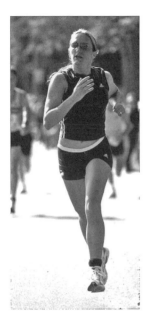

Negative foot speed can be eliminated by practicing the rule "foot-up, knee-up" when running. This means you should run with dorsiflexion and high-knee action. The hips should be slightly "thrust" forward.

The goal is for the foot to strike mid-foot, and not too high on the toes. And don't let these stride technique corrections make you lean the upper-body backwards, which happens sometimes when the flexibility isn't where it needs to be.

Endurance athletes running 5Ks, 10Ks and marathons should use dorsiflexion and land mid-foot during long distance runs. Notice the dorsiflexion used by Christa Walter (left) during a 5K race.

One of the best ways to improve speed is to improve flexibility. Performing the 10-Minute Stretching Routine (*Chapter 6*) four times a week will typically yield a four-inch gain in flexibility in four weeks.

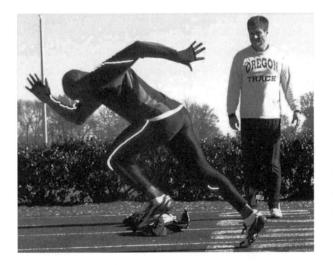

Lami Sama, sprinter from
Amsterdam, Netherlands
traveled 24 hours for individual
speed technique training

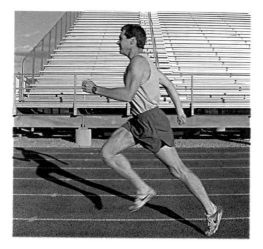

"The Sprint 8 amazingly increases my endurance very quickly. All distance runners should try this workout for a month, and they will permanently add it to their training,"
- **Leon Hoover, age 46**

"After being a competitive runner for over 36 years, I thought that there was little more that I could learn. I was totally wrong! Ready, Set, Go! Synergy Fitness has revolutionized my training and I can't thank Phil enough. I have lost body fat, gained energy and strength and I am running better than I have in years. Phil's book shows you how to incorporate his training methods into your bicycling, swimming, running or other cardiovascular workouts as well as maximize the benefit that you get from your strength workout. You owe it to yourself to read this book and start achieving all of the goals that you have always wanted to, but never been able to achieve."
- **Rich Drafter, Howtobefit Wellness Technology**

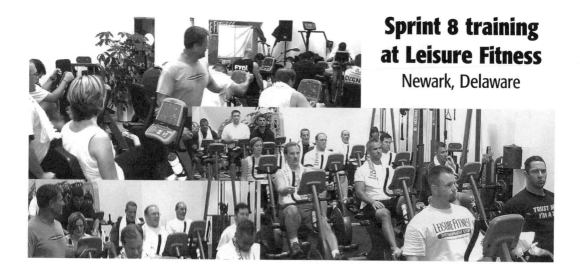

Sprint 8 training at Leisure Fitness
Newark, Delaware

Masters Track and Field

Runners over age 30, former athletes, and anyone wishing to use healthy competition for inspiration and additional motivation, should check out Masters Track and Field. Masters Track & Field is a division of USA Track & Field and has officially sanctioned events - www.MastersTrack.com, www.usatf.com, www.NationalMastersNews.com.

Conclusion

Throughout this book, high-intensity anaerobic exercise has been discussed because this type of fitness training can synergistically cut body fat, tone, and build muscle by increasing your body's natural fitness hormone.

Anaerobic exercise is the missing ingredient in most fitness plans. Whether your focus is losing weight, improving fitness, getting ready for the next season, anti-aging, or anti-middle-aging, anaerobic workouts are best at increasing exercise-induced growth hormone.

Anaerobic training is the toughest part of any fitness plan, but it is absolutely essential if you want the benefits of exercise-induced growth hormone. Give it a try. The winded condition at the end of a sprint may be uncomfortable during this 20-minute workout - but you'll love the results! And remember, when stepping up training intensity, increase slowly and progressively.

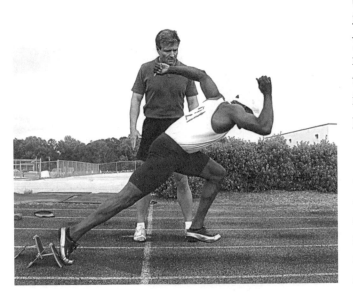

Phil Campbell working with Reginald Percival on an acceleration technique drill from starting blocks during an individual speed training session

9

Building Power with Plyometrics & E-Lifts

Power and strength are different. Power is strength in action. And developing explosive power with plyometrics will improve athletic performance.

High school athletes want fast-twitch muscle fiber to make the starting lineup. Olympians want fast muscle fiber to win the gold.

And everyone interested in getting the full benefit of exercise-induced growth hormone needs fast muscle fiber so high-intensity, anaerobic workouts can be performed throughout life.

Plyometric training is the champion at developing fast muscle fiber (IIa) and super-fast (IIx) muscle fiber.

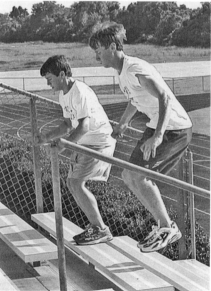

Adam Pipkin and Josh Liles perform
plyometric drills jumping up stadium seats

Plyometrics

"Plyometrics employs a quick, powerful movement involving a prestretch of the muscle, followed by a shortening, concentric muscular contraction, thus utilizing the stretch-shortening muscular cycle." (1993, Stretch-shortening drills for the upper extremities: theory and clinical application, J Orthop Sports Phys Ther, Wilk KE).

Plyometric drills typically involve jumping, skipping, and hopping but may be performed at lower intensities as long as the exercise is a fast movement involving a pre-stretched muscle followed by a quick and powerful shortening of a muscle (contraction).

In creating a plyometric drill, coaches take an important movement specific to a sport and create a drill that targets the movement. The drill develops the fast-twitch muscle fiber, along with training the central nervous system to react faster. Enhanced speed and power are the by-products of the plyometric drill.

Any sport needing increased running speed would need to have the common movements of running broken down and segmented into drills. The *High Knees* drill, for example, is a medium-intensity exercise designed to train the quads, hip flexors, and ankles to improve leg lift during running.

Butt Slaps train and develop the hamstrings to pull through the stride while running. These drills can be low, medium or high-intensity plyometric drills depending on the degree the exercise pushes the stretch-shortening cycle of the muscles involved.

Depending on how much jumping you put into these drills determines if they are to be called "form runs" or "plyometrics," and the goal is to make these drills plyometrics.

Karate Kicks, if they achieve the stretch-shortening cycle, are examples of low-intensity plyometrics.

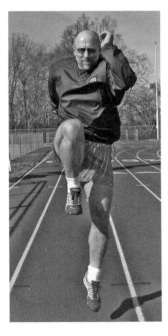

*John Blankenship, 1969-73 Middle Tennessee State University football wider-receiver, demonstrates how the **High Knees** drill can become a high-intensity plyometric drill by springing off the track with each step*

All Ages Benefit from Plyometrics

Children can increase bone density, strength, and power through plyometric jump drills (*Jumping improves hip and lumbar spine bone mass in prepubescent children: a randomized trial*, 2001, Fuchs).

Adolescent girls who participate in plyometric training increase bone density (*Effects of plyometric jump training on bone mass in adolescent girls*, 2000, Witzke).

Researchers demonstrate that regardless of age and physical condition, a total fitness plan should have exercises to improve power and develop fast-twitch muscle fiber. (Physio-pathologic aspects of aging– possible influence of physical training on physical fitness, 2000, Kostka).

ACL Knee Injury Warning:

Plyometric drills may aid in the prevention of ACL (anterior cruciate ligament) injuries - prevalent in certain sports. Drills must be performed with adequate warm-up and a gradual phase-in period because lateral movements may cause ACL injury.

Informative Websites:
http://orthoinfo.aaos.org
www.nlm.nih.gov/medlineplus/ency/article/001074.htm
www.aclprevent.com/pep_replacement.htm
www.aclsolutions.com

Premenopausal women maintain strength and power with plyometric training. Continued training also reduces several risk factors later in life (*Detraining reverses positive effects of exercise on the musculoskeletal system in premenopausal women*, 2000, Winters).

Senior men and women also need power and strength. Researchers report that the elderly are as responsive to strength training as younger adults (*Applied physiology of strength and power in old age*, 1994, Young). Clearly, strength and power do not need to be forgotten after the competitive days of youth are over. Many injuries in nursing homes occur from falls, which, perhaps, could be prevented with age-specific, functional strength training.

"This study indicates that a strength and plyometric program improved power endurance and speed over aerobic training only." (Changes evaluated in soccer-specific power endurance either with or without a 10-week, in-season, intermittent, high-intensity training protocol, 2003 May, J Strength Cond Res, Siegler J).

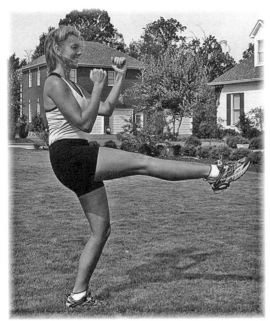

Plyometrics are performed by sets/reps similar to strength training. Conveniently, plyometric drills in the Ready, Set, Go! Fitness program can be performed almost anywhere.

Most of the plyometric drills in this chapter involve moving forward for 15 yards followed by a walk-back to the start for the recovery.

Personal trainer, Bambi LaFont, age 44, performs karate kicks and plyometric bounding

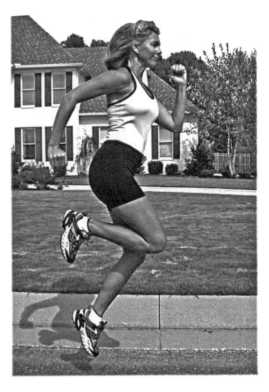

The following chart outlines the Plyometric workout that is programmed into the Strategic Fitness Plans in Chapter 11.

Power Building Plyometrics

Plyometric Kicks	Workout:
Front Karate Kicks	1 set / 10 kicks - each leg
Side Karate Kicks	1 set / 10 kicks
Back kicks	1 set / 10 kicks
Plyometric Drills	*(medium - high intensity)*
High Knees	1 to 2 sets / 15 yards
Butt Slaps	1 - 2 / 15 yds
Wall Slides	1 - 2 / 15 yds
Lunges (See *Note)	1 - 2 / 15 yds
Optional Plyometrics	*(high intensity)*
High Skips Bounding	1 / 15 yds

Beginning with standing karate kicks, perform one set of 10 karate kicks - front, side, and back as illustrated on the next three pages. Initially, make these drills low intensity and gradually increase the intensity so that the movements will be fast and involve the stretch-shortening cycle on each kick.

*Note - Lunges are included in the Ready, Set, Go! Fitness Plyometric Workout *even though this exercise is not technically a plyometric drill (unless a quick high-jump is added to the up phase).*

Lunges build strong leg muscles, and they are added to finish.

Karate Front Kicks

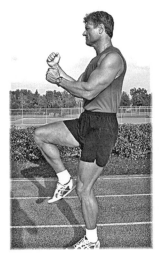

Start   Raise knee   Front kick, waist level

Note: Make karate kicks plyometric by engaging the stretch-shortening cycle of the muscle. The return of the leg after the kick needs to snap back as quickly as the kick itself

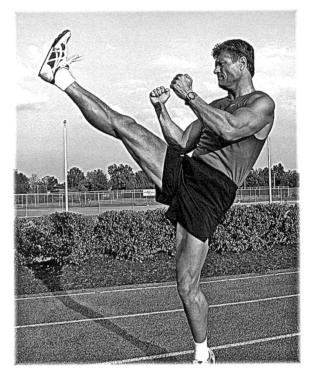

Advanced front kick

Karate Side Kicks

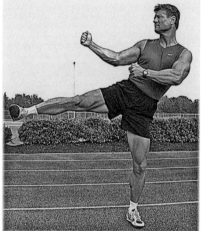

Start   Cock leg   Fire kick to waist level

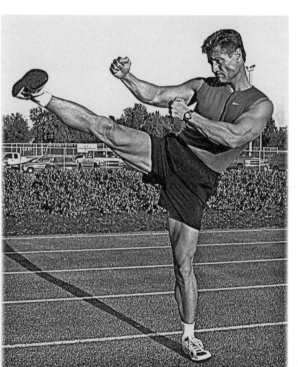

Advanced side kick

Karate Back Kicks

Start

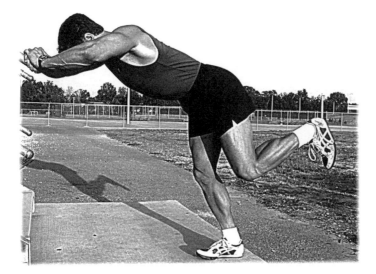

Back kick to waist level

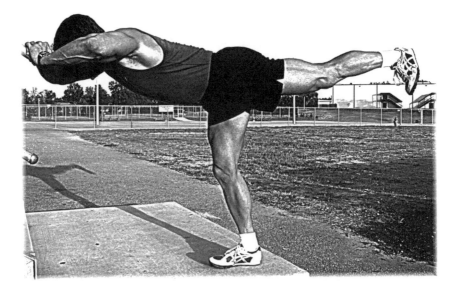

Dr. Douris Teaches Self Defense Against Aging

"Want to do something that's fun, different and good for self-defense, and good for long-term self-defense against disease, do martial arts," says researcher Dr. Peter Douris, Professor, Physical Therapy Department, New York Institute of Technology.

In a recent study, Dr. Douris reported that middle-aged martial art practitioners had developed greater aerobic capacity, balance, flexibility, muscle endurance, and strength, and less body fat than the sedentary group and martial arts can be considered *"an excellent form of exercise for the promotion of fitness in adults,"* (Fitness levels of middle aged martial art practitioners, 2004, Douris, P., British J Sports Med. 2004 Apr;38(2):143-7).

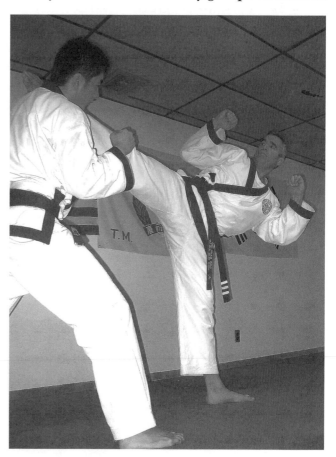

Dr. Douris believes adults of all ages should consider using karate-like sports for exercise. He says, *"It's not like judo, where you're doing a lot of flips and throws. You may fall down when you're 'free-sparring,' but there are men and women in martial arts classes that are 60 years old, and they get right back up."*

Douris, 49, is a 3rd degree dan (black belt) in two martial arts, Soo Bahk Do and Tae Kwon Do.

Dr. Peter Douris sparring with Dae Keun Kwon. Both are 3rd dan (3rd degree) in Soo Bahk Do, a Korean martial art

Plyometric Drills

Once the plyometric kicks have been completed, it is time to move to the medium-intensity, dynamic (moving forward) plyometric drills.

Initially, perform only one set of drills covering 10 yards. Progressively build to two sets of 15 yards with a walk-back recovery in between. This segment should only take 10 minutes initially and build to 20 minutes.

With all plyometric drills, there should be lots of explosive leg action (up and down) that achieves the stretch-shortening muscle cycle. However, the progress forward should be equal to the speed of walking.

For an advanced method of performing the plyometric drills, place a marker at every 5-yard point for the 15-yard drill. During the first 5 yards, move at a low-intensity rate with perfect form. During the second 5 yards, increase the intensity to full speed, but stay relaxed. For the final 5 yards, take the intensity all the way up and spring off the ground with every step.

High Knees

Run forward while raising knees high. Make sure the thigh of the raised knee is at least parallel to the track on each repetition.

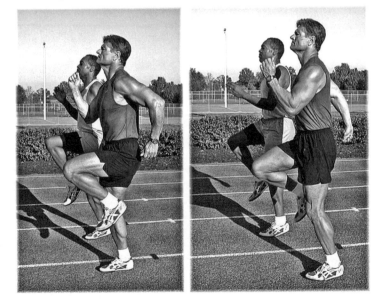

High Knees shown with my running partner, Nate Robertson

Butt Slaps

This drill is typically called *butt slaps* or *butt kickers*. Whatever the name, it's a great developer of fast-twitch leg muscles. This drill is especially valuable for the athletes wanting to improve speed. Run forward by raising the back foot as high as possible without raising the knee. Important: keep knees pointed downward during the entire drill.

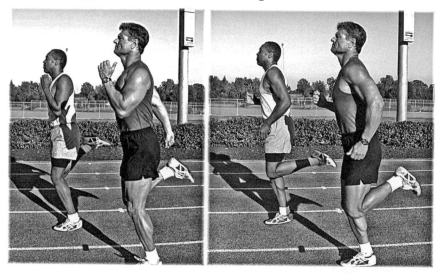

Don't get in a hurry with this drill. This is not a race forward. Move fast to activate the fast-twitch muscle in an aggressive up-and-down motion with your feet. The actual progress forward should be equal to the pace of walking.

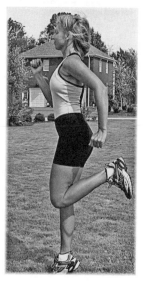

*Plyometrics may be easily
performed at home
in the yard*

Wall Slides

This drill has been called *wall slides, glass wall,* and *fast feet.* This drill is halfway between the *high knees* drill and the *butt slaps* drill. While moving forward, the knee is brought upward and high, while the foot is limited to coming up in a straight path directly under the body.

This drill is called "wall slides" because you visualize an imaginary wall (from head to toe) directly behind you as you move forward. See how the foot slides up the wall in the following illustration. Remember to make this drill plyometric by essentially jumping vigorously and springing off the track with each step.

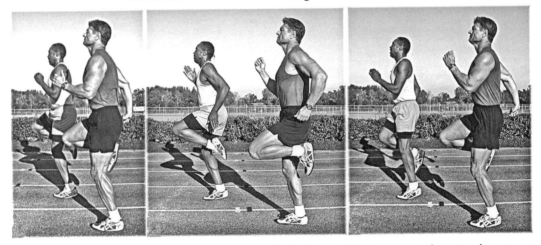

This is a great drill for athletes wanting to increase running speed because it teaches the "fly phase" of sprinting. This is the phase in sprinting that is considered upright running at "absolute speed." Athletes not trained in how to convert from the initial "drive phase" of running to "fly phase" will significantly deter speed in distances longer than 30 yards.

Arms should be locked at 90 degrees, moving *pocket to chin* level, and the foot should be striking the surface directly below the center of the body.

Lunges

Lunges are performed by taking steps forward at a slow-walking pace to finish this workout. With hands on hips, take a giant step forward and dip until the forward thigh becomes parallel with the track. Continue walking forward with the reaching lunge steps.

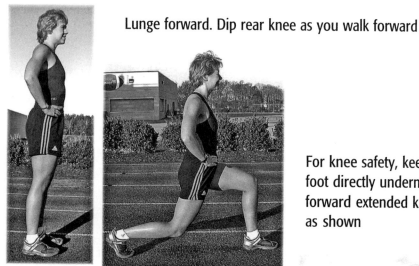

Lunge forward. Dip rear knee as you walk forward

For knee safety, keep the foot directly underneath the forward extended knee as shown

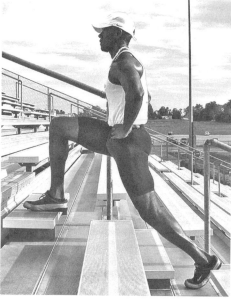

Advanced lunges can be performed by adding a plyometric jump while moving from the down to up position or by lunging up stadium steps as shown by Reginald Percival

High-intensity Plyometric Bounding

Plyometric bounding can be performed in many different ways. The Ready, Set, Go! Fitness method is easy. Remember how to skip? Just skip, except at the top of the skip - jump upward and as high as possible. Landing can be tough on the ankles, so before you add this high-intensity plyometric drill to your fitness plan, make sure you have been performing the basic plyometric workout for at least 90 days.

High Skips Bounding

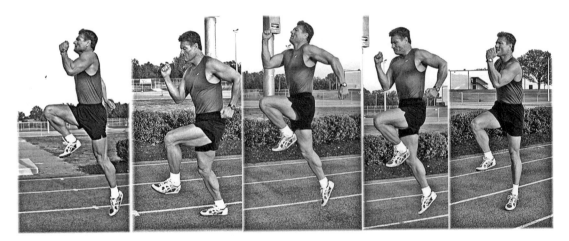

Scheduling Plyometric Drills

Plyometric drills should become a regular part of your fitness plan at least one day per week - beginning with Fitness Level Two. *E-Lifts* can be added to your strength training program to target fast-muscle fiber. And you can multi-task plyometric drills with an aerobic workout by limiting the recovery to 30 seconds between each drill.

Plyometrics help Ms. Fitness USA
Nicole Avellina

"Phil, the Sprint 8 is going to help to make me the next World Champion. Thank you so much!"
- **Nicole Avellina, Ms. Fitness USA**

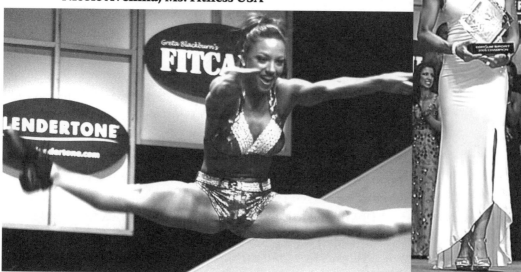

Nicole Avellina incorporates plyometrics, explosive E-Lifts strength training, the Sprint 8, and active-reflex stretching in her training and fitness competition preparation.

Based on the performance levels and conditioning necessary for Ms. Fitness competitions, personally, I consider Ms. Fitness competitions a sport because these women are athletes. And the training they perform is as comprehensive as it gets.

When looking at the national obesity issue from a societal viewpoint, there's agreement that the commitment to *fitness for a lifetime* must begin early in life, and continue through adolescence because it's difficult to reverse a history of inactivity.

It's for these reasons that I believe that Ms. Fitness competitions should become a high school sport. Judging these competitions is similar to the judging in gymnastics and cheering. More on Nicole Avellina at www.NicoleAvellina.com.

"Weightlifting performances and vertical jump power were correlated with type II fiber characteristics."
2003 Nov, *Muscle fiber characteristics and performance correlates of male Olympic-style weightlifters.*
J Strength Cond Res, Fry AC).

Why You Need E-Lifts in Your Training Plan

If you've been in the gym during the past few years, you've probably heard these strength training strategies tossed around; light weight / high reps and heavy weight / low reps. The newest strength training strategy on the block is Slow Reps, which refers to a slow moving repetition tempo. Think about doing a standard barbell curl in super-slow motion, and that's what Slow Reps look like.

I've been in the gym for 38 years and I've seen fitness fads and gimmicks come and go. And I've even seen some training gimmicks reinvented under different names, as if they were new revolutionary discoveries. New training techniques can be positive, particularly if they evolve from an established and proven system of training.

Plyometrics is a good example of the positive evolution of training methods.

Plyometrics take different forms, but these exercises are closely related to calisthenics that were used by coaches and drill sergeants during the 40s - 70s. Then some Russian engineers took calisthenics, applied some basic science for sports specific training, and evolved this form of exercise to a new level. Today we call these exercises plyometrics. Coaches use plyometrics worldwide to improve athletic performance by developing fast-twitch muscle fiber.

The evolution of plyometrics teaches us that it's important to challenge training methods and improve them when possible. On the positive side, the Slow Reps method reinforces the need to isolate muscle groups during strength training. Since Arthur Jones and Dr. Ellington Darden (www.drdarden.com) revolutionized the strength training scene in the 70s with high-intensity training (HIT), the principle of isolation has been one of the three key concepts in my strength-training programs.

Isolation means to train one muscle group completely by eliminating other groups that attempt to jump in and assist the targeted muscle group once those muscles get fatigued. This allows the muscle group to get more work, and the targeted muscles adapt to this training method by becoming bigger and stronger.

Isolation is an important training strategy and the Slow Reps method clearly helps to isolate targeted muscle groups. And that's positive, but Slow Reps can be limiting because muscles adapt. You can't be around an exercise physiologist very long without hearing the word "adaptation," because that's what muscles do. When muscles are trained, they adapt. Training slow develops slow-twitch muscle fiber, but it's necessary to train fast to reach fast-twitch fiber.

Slow reps, as well as the traditional lifting tempo of *up-on-two and down-on-four*, works slow muscle fiber. Again, that's positive because slow-twitch fiber is close to half of your muscle fiber (*Chapter 5*), but that leaves you with the other half of your muscle fiber decreasing in size and strength.

Now, if you plan on living life in slow motion, or play a sport where being slow is positive, then you may not want to add E-lifts to your training program. But if you want to work all of your muscle fiber, then just try E-lifts one time, and you'll know that this method is the real deal.

Will this method work for adults of all ages? Researchers report *yes* in a landmark , first-of-its-kind, new study led by Nathan De Vos:

Researchers show that plyometrics and weight training compliment each other in a total fitness model. (Weight and plyometric training: effects on eccentric and concern force production, 1996, Wilson).

> *Therefore, using heavy loads during explosive resistance training may be the **most effective strategy** to achieve simultaneous **improvements in muscle strength, power, and endurance in older adults**.*
>
> (Optimal load for increasing muscle power during explosive resistance training in older adults, J Gerontol A Biol Sci Med Sci. 2005 May;60(5):638-47, De Vos, NJ).

Professional athletes use explosives types of lifting because Olympic lifts are proven to yield better results in power than traditional power lifting (bench press, squat, and dead lift). Researchers show that 88 percent of US professional football coaches use Olympic lifting in their training and 94 percent use plyometric drills. *(Strength and conditioning practices of National Football League strength and conditioning coaches, 2001 Feb, J Strength Cond Res, Ebben W).*

The reason so many professional teams use explosive techniques in their strength training programs is simple. Superior results and a complete body of research shows that E-lifting yields better results in performance. Researchers report:

> *Results suggest that Olympic lifting can provide a significant advantage over power lifting in vertical jump performance changes. (Comparison of Olympic vs. traditional power lifting training programs in football players, 2004 Feb, J Strength Cond Res. Hoffman JR).*

E-Lifts are clearly superior for athletes, but what about the rest of us? E-Lifts again outperform other training methods. In a major new study, researchers show that older adults respond better to rapid-rate-of-force movements, and this type of training can be performed safely at older ages:

> *Progressive resistance training that incorporates rapid rate-of-force development movements may be safely undertaken in healthy older adults and results in significant gains in muscle strength, muscle power, and physical performance. Such improvements could prolong functional independence and improve the quality of life.*
> *(Improved physical performance in older adults undertaking a short-term programme of high-velocity resistance training. Gerontology. 2005 Mar-Apr;51(2):108-15, Henwood, TR).*

Another hot new study validates the fact that explosive lifting is the most successful training strategy for older adults:

Therefore, using heavy loads during explosive resistance training may be the most effective strategy to achieve simultaneous improvements in muscle strength, power, and endurance in older adults. *(Optimal load for increasing muscle power during explosive resistance training in older adults,* J Gerontol ABiol Sci Med Sci. 2005 May;60(5):638-47, De Vos, NJ).

I'm not talking about using light weight and moving through a set with a lot of quick up-and-down repetitions. I'm talking about using heavy weight and adding explosion during the movement away from the body. There's a big difference in performing repetitions quickly as opposed to explosively.

E-Lifting Mechanics

E-Lifting is short for *explosive lifting technique* and is an attempt to take the best from the world of Olympic Lifting — Clean & Jerk, Snatch — and the best from traditional lifting techniques used by bodybuilders and fitness trainers.

Simply adding an explosive movement on all push and press exercises will accomplish the fast-fiber training goal, which means you're working more muscle fiber than with slow movements, and that's why using E-Lifts yields better results. Muscle adapts to training; train fast to get fast, train slow and you're only using the slow-muscle fiber.

Exercises performed as a push or a press type of exercise are connected to muscle groups loaded with fast-twitch fiber. And these muscle groups require a fast, explosive tempo when pushing the resistance away from the body in order to reach the fast fiber. Examples of exercises would be bench press or any chest press type of machine, leg press, shoulder press, and even calf raises qualify as a push type of exercise.

Therefore, using heavy loads during explosive resistance training may be the most effective strategy to achieve simultaneous improvements in muscle strength, power, and endurance in older adults.
(Optimal load for increasing muscle power during explosive resistance training in older adults, J Gerontol A Biol Sci Med Sci. 2005 May;60(5):638-47, De Vos, NJ).

E-Lifting involves a brief, 1- to 2-second pause at the bottom of a lifting exercise. This will fully stretch the muscle and perhaps make the Slow Reps fans feel more comfortable with the technique. Then push the resistance with explosive thrust away from the body.

The down movement prior to the explosive thrust should be similar to the traditional weightlifting tempo of a 2 to 4-second pace.

For safety, there are two key points. There should be a warm-up set performed using the traditional lifting tempo of up-on-two, down-on-four. And you should fully extend the repetition all the way out on the push away from the body, but stop the explosive pushing at the 90 percent point to avoid injury to the elbows or knees. You don't stop at 90 percent, just stop pushing at 90 percent and fully extend.

Since 1970, I've worked with thousands of athletes and individuals in my Speed Camps and personal training. When it comes to strength training I have experimented with every new method that makes sense. I've found no other training method that comes close to getting these results from strength training. Not just for athletes preparing for the pro or college combines, but adults of all ages get superior results with E-Lifts.

Strength + Explosion = Results

Louie Simmons may not call his weight training program "E-Lifts," but his methods sound similar. Louie is a power lifter who squatted over 900 pounds at age 52. He was stronger at 52 than at 42, and stronger at 42 than at 32. His training plan builds strength.

His program consists of training four times a week - two days of upper body and two days of lower body. He also alternates a heavy day with an "explosive day." Strength training that includes explosive lifting yields positive results.

Bench Press E-Lifts

The E-Lift technique works well with push and press types of exercises like bench press, leg press, and shoulder press. Using the bench press as an example; lower the bar to your chest, which fully stretches this muscle group. Pause briefly (two counts), and explode the weight upward quickly and powerfully.

Extend arms fully during the rep but quit pushing at the 90 percent point. Explosive lifting works the fast muscle fiber that frequently goes untouched in most gyms.

"High-intensity progressive resistance training, in combination with moderate weight loss, was effective in improving glycemic control in older patients with type 2 diabetes."
(2002, High-intensity resistance training improves glycemic control in older patients with type 2 diabetes, Dunsta).

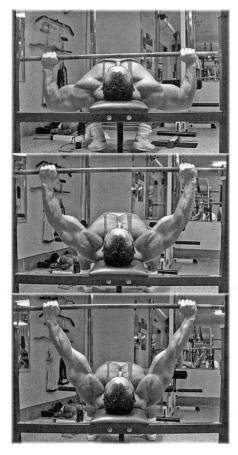

Control the descent of the bar until it touches the chest. Pause briefly in the lower position (two counts) before exploding up.

Explode upward.
Ease off the push at the 90 percent extension point.

Complete the full extension before the next rep.

Isshinryu 90 Percent Extension Principle for E-Lifts

The founder of Isshinryu Karate, Master Tatsuo Shimabuku (1906–1975), designed his form of marital arts to be a lifelong method of training by taking into consideration the risk of injury associated with fast, hard, full extension of the legs and arms during kicks and punches.

To prevent injury and increase power, the karate master developed a rule that should also be applied to training involving E-Lifts.

Master Shimabuku declared that all Isshinryu Karate punches and kicks would be limited to 90 percent extension. Applying this same principle with E-Lifts should help avoid injury while achieving the benefits of fast-twitch muscle development.

The key is to extend the arms (or legs) at the end of a repetition to 100 percent extension; just quit pushing at the 90 percent extension point so joints don't get over-extended.

Use Heathy Competition for Motivation

Placing yourself in a competition can be a wise self-motivation fitness improvement strategy. For women, the Ms. Fitness program is a wonderful invention. Training for fitness competitions requires a comprehensive approach consistent with the Ready, Set, Go! Fitness philosophy. Ms. Fitness competitors train for strength, flexibility, endurance, speed, coordination, balance, and about everything else that's positive for the body.

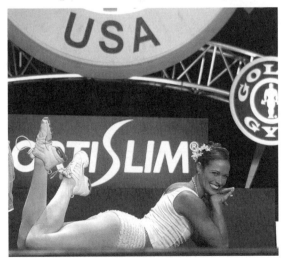

Large health improvement companies like CortiSlim are seeing the value of Ms. Fitness training, and are sponsoring events in new states every year - www.msfitness.com.

Sarah Harding, Ms. Fitness USA 2006

As a professional acrobat and All-American gymnast, I was excited to learn so many new tips on health and fitness at Greta Blackburn's Fit Camp. I especially loved reading guest speaker, Phil Campbell's book, "Ready, Set, GO!"

The Sprint 8 workouts are extremely efficient and beneficial to any athlete. They supplement my training and helped me get in the best shape of my life. I highly recommend Sprint 8 to anyone who wants to look and feel younger. The best part about it is the workouts are so efficient. You don't have to spend hours in the gym. You just have to challenge yourself to get faster. I love the fact that I can set new goals and feel younger with every stride!"

- **Sarah Harding, Ms. Fitness USA 2006**

www.sarahhardingfitness.com

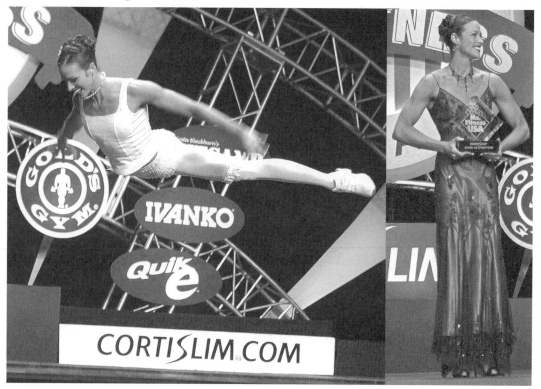

Photographs by Sami Vaskola

Hang Cleans for Power

Hang Cleans are slightly different from the Olympic version of *Power Cleans,* which begin at the floor and move up to the finish position in one movement.

Power Cleans have been modified over the years for safety. The modified version, *Hang Cleans,* begins just below the waist.

Extra caution needs to be taken with this lift, even for well-trained athletes. The initial movement from the floor to the start position needs to be performed with a straight back as shown (right) to avoid injury.

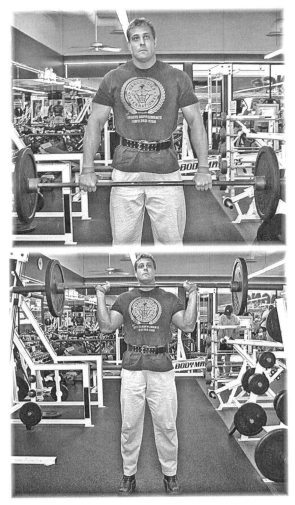

Hang Cleans and Olympic lifts are great for building power, however, there can be problems with these lifts. The main issue is that many younger athletes have been injured performing Olympic lifts because they do not yet have the muscular structure to support this type of lifting.

Personally, being over age 50, I cannot manage the weight necessary for these strenuous lifts. However, using the E-Lifts technique on traditional strength training exercises works well for me, and the athletes that I train.

Jason McCarver demonstrates hang cleans (front view)

Wearing support belts may be helpful when performing Olympic lifts, but this issue is controversial. Some trainers argue that if you need a belt to support lifting, you are using too much weight. Researchers report:

> *Wearing abdominal belts raises intramuscular pressure of the erector spine muscles and appears to stiffen the trunk. Assuming that increased intramuscular pressure of the erector spine muscles stabilizes the lumbar spine, wearing abdominal belts may contribute to the stabilization during lifting exertions. (Effects of abdominal belts on intraabdominal pressure, intramuscular pressure in the erector spinae muscles and myoelectrical activities of trunk muscles."* (Clin Biomech, 1999 Feb, Miyamoto K).

The Level Five Fitness Plan (for advanced athletes) in Chapter 11 includes Olympic and power lifting one day a week. For the other four levels, E-Lift techniques achieve the goals of working fast-muscle fiber when strength training.

Back straight   Start   Upward thrust

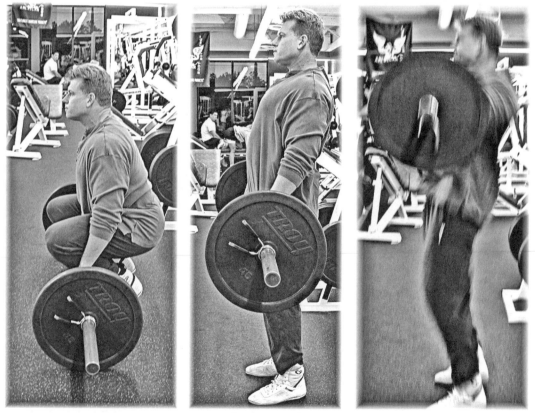

Dr. Don Buchanan demonstrates hang cleans (side view)

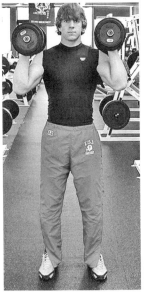

Push Press

Push press resembles the Olympic jerk lift. The first movement is to bend the knees as shown, then explode the dumbbells (or barbell) upward. Quit pushing at the 90 percent extension point so you don't over-extend your elbow joints.

It's good to pause (briefly) between each press to regain balance. This is a total body exercise, so come off your heels as you explode upward.

Start

Lower the body and explode the weight to 90 percent extension.

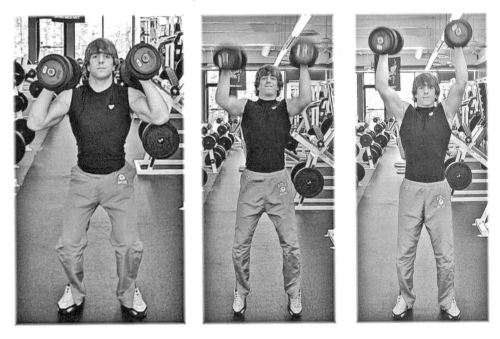

Randy Sheffield, All-Regional Defensive and All-State football player, demonstrates push press

Clean and Jerk

The Clean and Jerk is an Olympic lift consisting of two parts. The Clean, which gets the weight to the chest, is followed by the Jerk. The Jerk aspect of the lift is performed by quickly pressing the weight overhead while splitting the legs.

This advanced lift can be dangerous if it's not performed correctly. Only Level Five athletes should perform this exercise. Push Presses may be substituted for this lift.

Kirk Pafford demonstrates the
Clean and Jerk Olympic lift

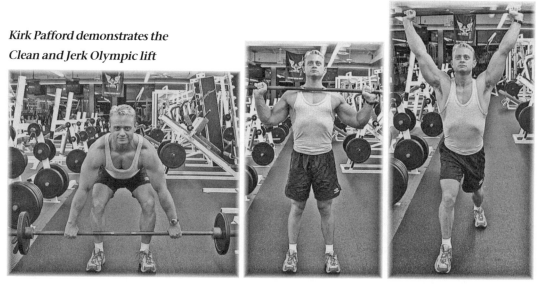

Start   First lift (Clean)   Finish lift (Jerk)

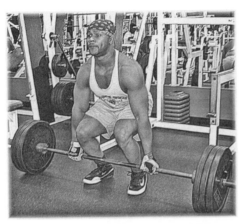

Dead Lift

The dead lift is an advanced power lift that can be very productive. Some trainers recommend a support belt for safety, and some others believe that if it's heavy enough to use a belt, then it's too heavy to lift with a belt.

Use the reverse grip on one hand and keep the back straight as the pull upward is made. Terrance Copeland demonstrates the correct form for a power dead lift.

Initial pull upward
keep the back straight

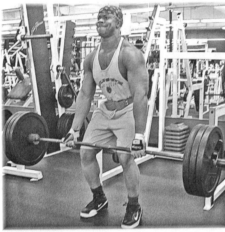

Important - Keep lower back straight

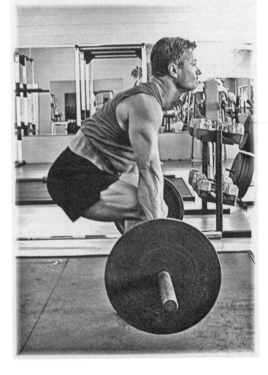

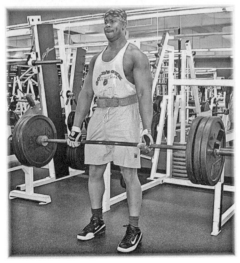

Fitness Competition Training

Fitness routines used in women's fitness competitions target strength, power, flexibility, endurance, and anaerobic development. There should be more encouragement for women and men to participate in this type of comprehensive training and competition.

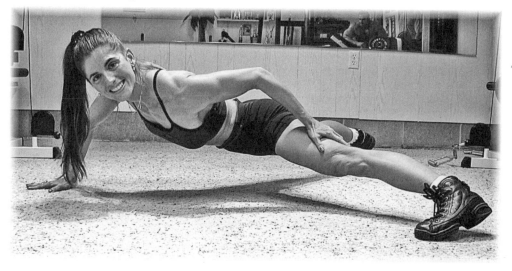

Photographs by Kathy Campbell

Kate Shelby, national fitness competition winner, practices her fitness routine

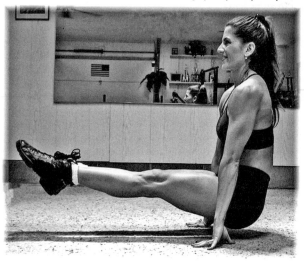

Conclusion

Performing plyometric drills, Olympic lifting and the E-Lifts technique discussed in this chapter will develop fast-twitch muscle fiber, which is essential in performing anaerobic HGH releasing exercise for a lifetime.

The following chapter, *Tactical Strength Training*, adds the weight-training component to the Ready, Set, Go! Fitness program.

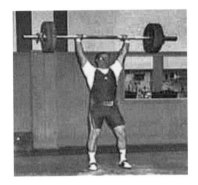

Ron Summers, age 52, finishes a 286 lb Clean & Jerk to place second in the National Masters Olympic Lifting Championships.
He is a three-time national masters shot put champion.

Ready, Set, Go! Synergy Fitness is a great book for anyone wanting to improve their fitness and health. The book is loaded with useful information and the programs are clear and easy to follow. - **Ron Summers**

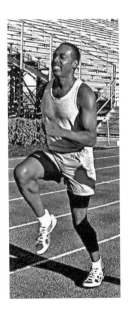

High Knees demonstrated by Nate Robertson

10

Tactical Strength Training

Strength training with weights or other resistance equipment is essential in achieving the goals of the Ready, Set, Go! Fitness program by building a strong body that can handle Sprint 8 types of anaerobic exercise for a lifetime.

Adding lean muscle through strength training will increase "resting metabolism," and this creates additional synergy in your body to further reduce body fat (2001, Rennie).

Whether it's weightlifting in a large chain fitness center, or a convenient workout at home, strength training is necessary, and it has many wonderful synergistic benefits.

New research shows that we need to change the way we think about strength training. In a new, first-of-its-kind study, the research team led by Nathan De Vos concludes:

> Using heavy loads during explosive resistance training may be the **most effective strategy** to achieve simultaneous **improvements in muscle strength, power, and endurance in older adults.**
> (Optimal load for increasing muscle power during explosive resistance training in older adults, J Gerontol A Biol Sci Med Sci. 2005 May;60(5):638-47, De Vos, NJ).

This simply means that we need to train like athletes all of our lives, not just when we are young. Of course,

Researchers at the University of Maryland show that strength training improves endurance. (Effects of strength training on lactate thresholds and endurance performance, 1991, Marcinik).

"High-intensity free weight-based training for frail elders appears to be as safe as lower intensity training but is more effective physiologically and functionally."
(Physiological and Functional Responses to Low-Moderate Versus High-Intensity Progressive Resistance Training in Frail Elders. J Gerontol A Biol Sci Med Sci. 2004 May, Seynnes O).

training needs to be modified for age, conditioning and training experience, but it needs to reach for productive, high-intensity levels. As you see the new research presented in this chapter, I hope you will make the commitment, no matter what your age, to begin training to build strength.

If you're female and over age 40, you must begin lifting weights! If you're in the nursing home, you must begin exercising to build strength! It's never too late to start.

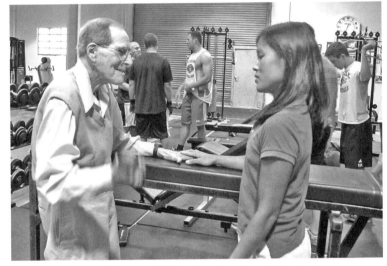

Max Riekes, age 97, having fun strength training with trainer Paula Chan, MS, PT, ATC (photo by Lex Ebbibk)

Adding New Muscle Makes Your Body a Fat-Burning Machine

The most efficient way to permanently lose excess body fat, according to researchers, is to implement a "diet with exercise" strategy. The idea of losing body fat without a strategy of developing muscle is not effective.

Researchers show that maintaining and adding muscle through strength training synergistically increases *metabolic rate, and this enhances your body's ability to reduce fat during rest* (Physical activity, overweight, and obesity, 2000, Stromme).

Strength training is a major component of the Ready, Set, Go! Fitness program. Regardless of your age or physical condition, training for strength and muscle development should be a part of your fitness plan. You can join a fitness center in your area, purchase a home strength trainer, or even get a set of free weights at a yard sale, but strength training needs to be in your fitness plan.

Weight Training Principles

Weightlifting and other forms of strength training following the principles discussed in this chapter will help you build the type of body it takes to handle anaerobic exercise that will release HGH. Some strength training exercises may actually reach the HGH-release benchmarks discussed in Chapter 1; muscle-burn (lactic acid), oxygen debt (winded), adrenal release (slightly painful), and increased body temperature (sweating).

Applying the following three principles of successful weight training will help you achieve higher exercise intensities and yield more benefits from your strength training program.

Fitness training, "substantially reduces obesity and insulin resistance." (Reduction in obesity and related comorbid conditions after diet-induced weight loss or exercise-induced weight loss in men, Ross, 2000). *Research subjects that did not lose weight during the research did lose body fat in the abdominal area.*

PRINCIPLES FOR SUCCESSFUL WEIGHT TRAINING

1. Isolation - of the muscle group being exercised

2. Exhaustion - of the muscles being worked during every set

3. Aerobic Recovery - Only rest briefly between sets (1 minute is ideal, 2 minutes maximum)

"Testosterone and growth hormone (GH) concentrations were significantly elevated." (2003 Nov, Effect of muscle oxygenation during resistance exercise on anabolic hormone response, Med Sci Sports Exerc, Hoffman JR).

Isolation

Isolating a muscle group during strength training makes a huge difference in the results you'll receive. Isolation of the muscle being worked makes you zone in and target the specific muscle, and this helps to define the goal of the exercise. And that leads to better results.

This principle means to isolate only one target muscle group that you are training. The hard part is to position the exercise to minimize any other muscle groups from assisting the targeted muscle.

Other muscle groups try to assist as the targeted muscle becomes fatigued, especially at the end of a set. If you allow other muscles to assist, the impact of training is decreased. This is the most difficult aspect of weight training technique. You should focus on not allowing other muscles to assist when the targeted muscle becomes fatigued.

For example, countless times I have talked with individuals, even serious bodybuilders and professional athletes, who cannot seem to build their biceps. This is an easy fix! Invariably, bicep curls were being performed with the wrists bent toward the body rather than straight. This positions the forearms to do much of the work, rather than the biceps. They thought they were working their biceps, and they were . . . some, but not enough to get results.

One aspect of the **ISOLATION PRINCIPLE** dictates keeping the wrist straight (and even slightly bending the wrist backwards during curls). Positioning the biceps this way prevents the forearms from assisting, thereby isolating the biceps. The biceps to do the work - and receive the full benefit of the exercise.

Correct - wrist straight.
Isolation is on bicep, not forearm

Incorrect - wrist bent in. Bicep not isolated, and the forearm is doing much of the work

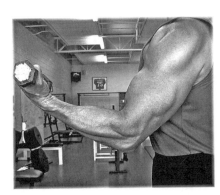
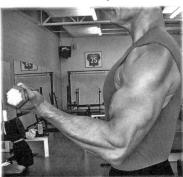

The Isolation Principle is also involved in the "free weights vs. machines" debate. It is argued that *absolute* isolation of the muscle with machines keeps the stabilizer muscles (muscles that stabilize the joints) from engaging, and therefore, free weights are better.

I don't think any trainer who has experienced the benefits of isolating muscle groups during strength training feels you should not work the stabilizers. The trainers that use the stabilizer argument for a "free weights only" training strategy will generally not use cables. And cable exercises clearly target the stabilizers much more than free weights.

The truth is that stabilizer muscles are extremely important. These muscles help provide fundamental balance for the body. The issue comes down to how best to work the stabilizers. And that depends on your training goals. If your goal is Olympic lifting, then you need to perform Olympic lifts and train as specifically as possible for the movements in your sport. And you may not need cable exercises, balance boards or strength training machines.

However, if building and toning muscle is your goal, then a comprehensive training approach, which may include free weights, machines, and cables can provide synergistic training benefits. The strength training strategy in this book is to target the stabilizers during Finishing Exercises with cable exercises and target the three muscle fiber types within large muscle groups by isolating the targeted muscle with Primary Exercises.

It's important to remember that *functional strength training* is for the way you live, and it produces meaningful results. Whether your life has you using joints, ligaments, and muscles to lift kids, or life has you pushing around linebackers, it's important to train for the activities and movements in your life. Life moves. It's not stationary. It's dynamic.

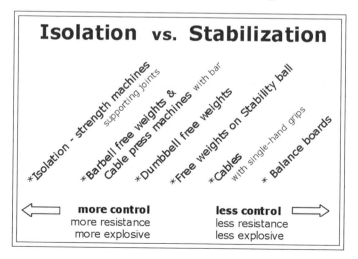

Researchers show that multiple sets per body part produce greater strength gains than one set per body part.
(Borst, 2001).

"These findings are consistent with the literature for the bench-press exercise and indicate that 1-minute rest intervals are sufficient for recovery between attempted lifts during 1RM (one-rep max) testing or training for the free-weight back squat." (Effect of rest interval length on repeated 1 repetition maximum back squats. 2003 Nov. J Strength Cond Res. Matuszak ME).

Exhaustion

Exhaustion of the muscle group during every set must occur - or don't count the set (and actually repeat the set). This is a good rule to follow and will yield great results. But this is also a tough rule to follow. If you have not experienced "going to failure" during every set, it can be fatiguing and the lactate can burn the muscles - but it's worth the effort.

Typically, individuals limit an exercise to a prescribed number of repetitions (reps) when more could be done. For example, *"Chest: Incline bench press, 3/10"* on a fitness plan means the *chest* is the targeted muscle group, *incline bench press* is the exercise, and the training plan is *3 sets of 10 repetitions* with a 1-minute rest between sets - and most will stop at 10 reps on each of the 3 sets.

Stopping at 10 reps isn't exhaustion! Exhaustion on every set means to keep going until you can't do anymore reps. Don't stop at 10 reps simply because the plan states "3/10." The "3/10" is a generalized goal to get you in the ballpark of where you were the last time you performed the exercise.

The **EXHAUSTION PRINCIPLE** dictates squeezing out 11 or 12 reps, or more if possible. If you can perform 13 to 15 reps, it's time to increase resistance by adding 5 to 10 pounds during the next workout.

Gary Riekes, founder of the Riekes Center in Menlo Park, California says it best, *"training to failure is success."*

Aerobic Recovery
One-Minute Rest Between Sets is Ideal

Make weight training an aerobic workout. You can multi-task aerobic exercise and resistance training simultaneously by only resting briefly between sets.

Ideal rest between sets is a 1-minute rest. A 1.5-minute

rest is acceptable, and 2 minutes should be the maximum.

Multi-tasking strength training with cardio not only saves time, it also produces great results.

Not effective is the style of weight training where an individual performs a set, stops at 10 reps (when 15 could have been performed), and rests several minutes between sets. This will not increase HGH or burn many calories.

It's okay to take a 2-minute rest between training body parts during split-training routines. However, while working a body part - stay focused on the 1-minute rest between sets.

On days when I feel like I need more than a 1-minute rest between sets, I silently say to myself, "Ready, Set, GO!" then start the set. This is a personal mental trigger to "get tough, get focused, and get going" and with intensity I start the set.

Target Zones and E-Lifts

The strength-training exercises in this chapter have *Target Zones* within every muscle group being worked. The exercises target slow-twitch muscle fiber, and E-Lifting techniques (*illustrated in Chapter 9*) target the fast-twitch muscle fiber and should be used on all push and press exercises once you reach Fitness Level Two.

Fatiguing your muscles, raising body temperature, and achieving muscle burn are the goals during every set.

SYNERGY FITNESS STRATEGY 9
During strength training, isolate muscles being worked, train every set to exhaustion, aerobically

Therefore, using heavy loads during explosive resistance training may be the most effective strategy to achieve simultaneous improvements in muscle strength, power, and endurance in older adults. (Optimal load for increasing muscle power during explosive resistance training in older adults, 2005, J Gerontol A Biol Sci Med Sci. 2005 May;60(5):638-47, De Vos, NJ

"It is concluded that heavy resistance exercise is safer when performed while the subject breathes with a ... slow exhalation during the concentric contraction (push up or out movement)."

NOTE: Blood pressure increased during lifting to 198/175 with the slow exhale method, whereas holding the breath (Valsalva technique) increased blood pressure to 311/284 during the concentric lift. (Influence of breathing technique on arterial blood pressure during heavy weight lifting. Arch Phys Med Rehabil. 1995 May, Narloch JA).

The Ultimate Weightlifting Question: What's Best?
High Reps/Low Weight, or Low Reps /Heavy Weight?

The answer to this question is . . . yes! Both methods are effective. The underlying principle is in the "intensity of the exercise" not a precise number of repetitions.

Researchers show that eight reps (at 80 percent of an individual's one-rep maximal lift) versus 16 reps (at 40 percent of maximal lift) obtain equal results in women during six months of training (*Musculoskeletal responses to high- and low-intensity resistance training in early postmenopausal women, 2000, Bemben*).

The answer to this question may be different for experienced athletes, however. Researchers report: "Athletes training at 80 percent of their one-rep max had significantly greater strength improvements than athletes training below (this intensity) for both bench press and squat" (*Strength changes during an in-season resistance-training program for football.* J Strength Cond Res. 2003 Feb, Hoffman JR).

Breathing During Resistance Training

The rule on breathing during resistance training is simple. **Exhale when the repetition is the most difficult.**

Inhale on the return movement. Example: On press type exercises such as the bench press or shoulder press, exhale on the press *up* (or press *out*) movements and inhale while lowering the weight.

On pull downs or cable rows, exhale on the pull *down* (or pull *in*) movement and inhale as you release the weight.

Fitness Center Membership?

Strength training can be performed with resistance in many forms besides weightlifting in a fitness center. Time-crunched adults may not have the time to drive to a gym. If you are self-disciplined, you *can* make a fitness plan work at home.

Dr. Keith Williams, a physician with a full-time Ob-Gyn practice, the chairman of deacons at his church, and an active parent of four children, finds four hours a week for the Level Two Fitness Plan.

He uses inexpensive free weights, a bench, and has a 70-yard course marked in his front yard for his Sprint 8 Workouts.

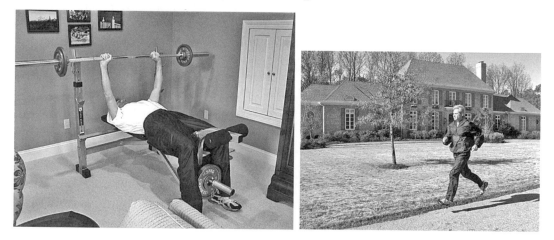

A fitness center membership will provide a certain amount of peer pressure that can be positive. Research shows that there is an important social aspect associated with a fitness center membership. And these relationships are sometimes very effective in maintaining consistency.

There's more information available about fitness centers at: www.HEALTHCLUBS.com and www.fitcommerce.com.

Researchers at the University of Maryland show that strength training improves endurance. *(Effects of strength training on lactate thresholds and endurance performance, 1991, Marcinik).*

"How am I motivated," may be a necessary question to ask yourself concerning a fitness center membership. Making fitness training convenient is an important factor in maintaining a long-term fitness program. And this is why so many people are purchasing home cardio equipment and home gyms. There is only so much time in a day, and eliminating a few minutes of drive time can mean the difference in getting in a workout that day, or not.

If you enjoy social relationships, consider a gym membership, walking club, running club, fitness club, or you could start your own Ready, Set, Go! Fitness Group and recruit some friends and colleagues to begin with you.

If you respond to competition, place yourself in a competitive environment - check out Masters Track and Field on the Internet www.masterstrack.com, www.usatf.org or other masters' sports competitions.

You can find a way to make this happen!

Repetition Tempo

With the exception of explosive E-Lifts on push and press movements, the basic tempo for weightlifting repetitions should be approximately 2 seconds going up, and 3 to 4 seconds going down. Newcomers to fitness training should begin at the Level One Fitness Plan, and the tempo should not be performed at the explosive E-Lifts tempo until moving to Fitness Level Two and above.

Even at advanced levels, pulling-type exercises should be at a slightly slower rate - pull in on a count that lasts 2 to 3 seconds and the release should last 3 to 4 seconds (*pull downs, cable pulls, and curls*).

Whole or Split-Body Training?

"Whole-body" strength training is prescribed for Fitness Levels One and Two. *Split-body routines* begin at Fitness Level Three because the work load of this Level with high-intensity training is too great to be performed during a single day.

Whole vs. Split-Body Training Comparisons

After 20 weeks of weight training for newcomers

Results:	Whole-body	Split-body
Decrease in Body fat	4.9%	1.7%
Leg Muscle Increase	4.1%	2.6%
Overall Muscle Increase	(1.1%) *loss*	(1.3%) *loss*

"Results demonstrate that for recreationally trained individuals 3 sets of training are superior to 1 set for eliciting maximal strength gains." (Three sets of weight training superior to 1 set with equal intensity for eliciting strength. J Strength Cond Res. 2002 Nov, Rhea MR).

During the first five months of strength training, research shows (for young healthy women), that whole-body routines slightly outperform split-body routines (*Comparison of whole and split weight training routines in young women*, 1994, Calder). Whole-body routines are preferred for newcomers to strength training.

Weight Training is Anti-Aging

"Exercise programs designed to improve muscle strength are recommended for older individuals as an effective countermeasure to the sarcopenia (frailty) of old age." (Effects of exercise training in the elderly, 1995, Proc Nutr Soc, Fielding RA).

Weight training is beneficial for all ages. Even women with chronic heart failure (CHF) benefit from lifting weights. Researchers studied the impact of strength training on 16 older women with chronic heart failure.

Results: Exercise was "well-tolerated" and strength was improved by 8.8 percent. **Endurance improved by 66 percent**, and type I muscle fiber increased 16 percent during the 10-week study period (2001, Pu).

In another study, 40 adults, average age 69, were divided into two groups and completed either six months of weight training or six months of endurance training.

Researchers determined that the endurance-trained group improved "oxidative capacity" (the body's ability to supply oxygen to the blood) by 31 percent, but **the resistance-trained group improved 57 percent**. The weight-training group also experienced a 10 percent increase in muscle size (*Large energetic adaptations of elderly muscle to resistance and endurance training*, 2001, Jubrias).

Max Riekes, age 97, trains with weights four times a week

The results of these studies are important, if not profound. First, strength training was successful in producing extremely positive results. The endurance group made remarkable improvement, and the resistance-training group almost doubled those results. Don't drop the cardio, just add weight training to your fitness program.

Strength training performed by older men and women produces many wonderful benefits: it increases endurance, normalizes blood pressure, reduces insulin resistance, reduces body fat, increases resting metabolic rate, reduces pain in knee joints, and most importantly, weight training reduces the risk of falls, which can be deadly in older populations (*Strength training in elderly effects on risk factors for age related diseases*, 2000, Hurley).

Middle-aged and older men participating in strength training research, experience "significant" gains in strength and power in 16 weeks of training. (Effects of strength training on muscle power and serum hormones in middle-aged and older men, 2000, Izquierdo).

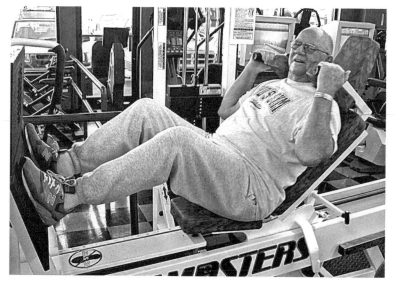

Freddie Hutchinson strengthening his legs with Leg Press

Strength Training for Children?

Strength training for children has been long debated. New research provides the answers.

Researchers at LSU Medical School show that even obese children (ages 7 to 12) benefit from resistance training.

After one year of resistance training, children in the study "significantly" reduced fat. Resistance training also produced a positive exercise retention factor for the children (*Safety, feasibility, and efficacy of a resistance training program in preadolescent obese children*, 2000, Sothern).

What do pediatricians say about children lifting weights? The American Academy of Pediatrics issued a new position. The 2001 report cites the many benefits of strength training for teenagers and even preadolescents. Earlier concerns of injuries to the wrist and back were reported as "largely preventable by avoiding improper lifting techniques, maximal lifts, and improperly supervised lifts."

Does weightlifting stunt growth in children? No, reports the AAP. "Strength training programs do not seem to adversely affect linear growth" (AAP citing "*The effects of a twice-a-week strength training program for children*," Faigenbaum, 1993).

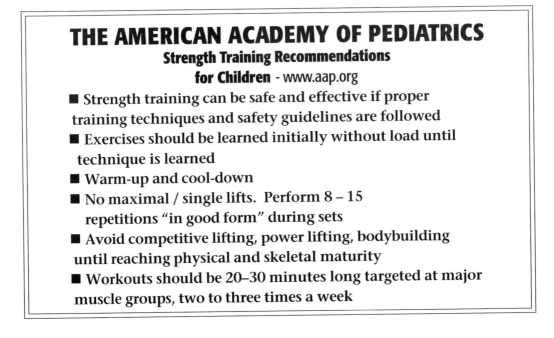

THE AMERICAN ACADEMY OF PEDIATRICS
Strength Training Recommendations
for Children - www.aap.org

- Strength training can be safe and effective if proper training techniques and safety guidelines are followed
- Exercises should be learned initially without load until technique is learned
- Warm-up and cool-down
- No maximal / single lifts. Perform 8 – 15 repetitions "in good form" during sets
- Avoid competitive lifting, power lifting, bodybuilding until reaching physical and skeletal maturity
- Workouts should be 20–30 minutes long targeted at major muscle groups, two to three times a week

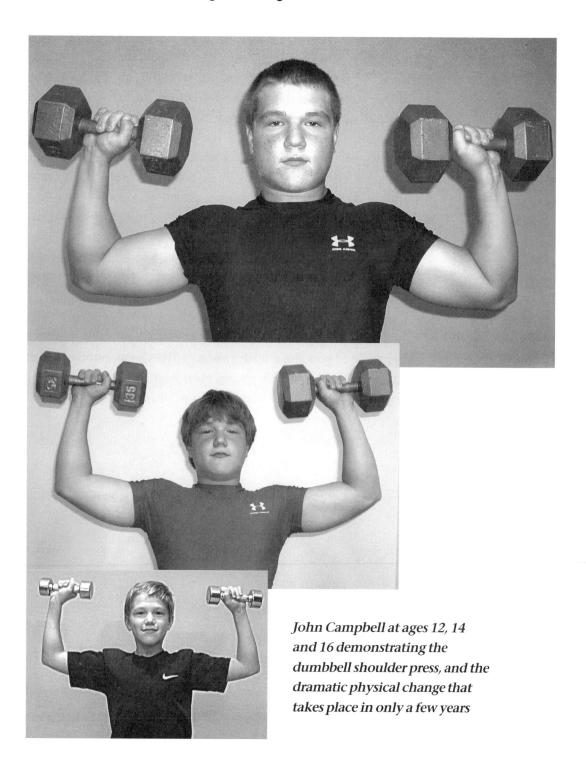

John Campbell at ages 12, 14 and 16 demonstrating the dumbbell shoulder press, and the dramatic physical change that takes place in only a few years

Use Training to Reach Youth

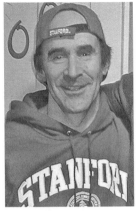

The youth mentoring program that Gary Riekes offers at the Riekes Center (named after his mother) in Menlo Park, California reaches youth where they are: fitness training, sports, nature studies, and creative arts.

This sports/fitness center not only has a full compliment of everything a fitness buff or pro could want – several pro athletes train here daily – the center even has a hands-on film/recording studio for those interested in learning more about the film and music industries.

How many teens would like to be a sports, film, or rock star? The Riekes Center knows how to reach teens! And they know how to train them to mentor others from knowledge gained at the center.

Gary Riekes, founder of the Riekes Center in Menlo Park, CA plays basketball with high school athletes training to improve performance **www.riekes.com**

This program is the most successful mentoring model I've seen. If you work with youth (YMCA or a church group) and you want to reach young men and women, you owe it to yourself to see the Riekes Center mentoring model.

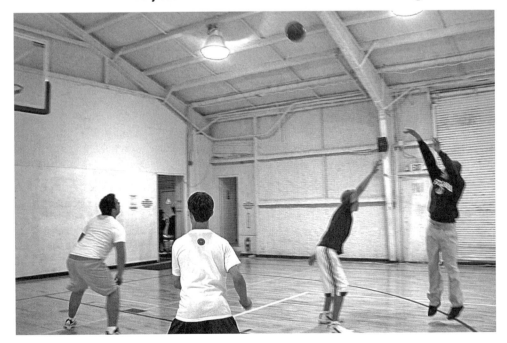

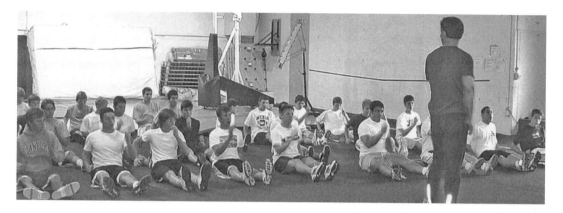

Teaching arm mechanics during Speed Camp at the Riekes Center

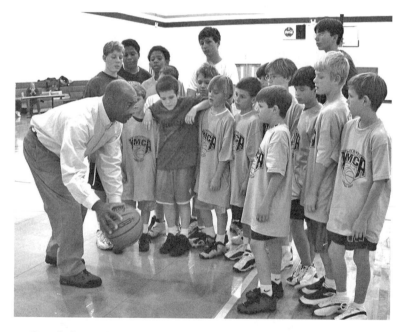

Coach Larry Jones, volunteer coach for over 25 years, uses
positive teaching techniques while coaching children

"A moderate-intensity weight training program increased strength and fat-free mass and decreased body fat in normal-weight young women. Favorable changes in body composition were obtained without restricting food intake." (Weight training increases fat-free mass and strength in untrained young women. J Am Diet Assoc. 1998 Apr, Cullinen K).

The basic Push Up is an example of using the body weight for sports-specific exercise resistance.

Some children may be unable to use their body weight in this fashion. If this is the case, the child may actually need to use weight training at home with lighter weight (perhaps much less than body weight) and high repetitions to build to the point where body weight resistance can be used.

Christine Campbell demonstrates the Push Up

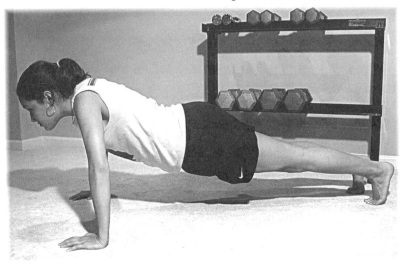

Personal Trainer: Do You Need One?

Personal trainers - if they are qualified, experienced (with your age group), motivated and motivating - can make positive things happen like help jump-start a fitness plan, or assist you through a training plateau.

How do you select a personal trainer? At your fitness center, ask friends who have used a personal trainer. Don't make the decision on the first name you hear. Spend some time making your decision.

Once you have someone in mind, talk to a couple of clients and ask about training philosophy, age group experience, time commitments, certification, and the amount of attention given during training. Be sure that the trainer uses a comprehensive Ready, Set, Go! Fitness type approach.

SOURCES FOR CERTIFIED PERSONAL TRAINERS

AAAI/ISMA
American Aerobics Association International & International Sports Medicine Association - www.aaai-ismafitness.com

AFAA Aerobics and Fitness Association of America - www.afaa.com

AFPA - www.afpafitness.com

AFTA Health & Fitness
www.aftacertification.com (Excellent Web site)

American Council on Exercise - www.acefitness.org

IDEA Health and Fitness Association - www.IDEAfit.com

IFPA International Fitness Professionals - www.ifpa-fitness.com

ISSA International Sports Sciences Association - www.issaonline.com

National Council of Strength and Fitness - www.ncsf.org

National Federation of Professional Trainers - www.nfpt.com

NESTA - www.nestacertified.com

*HMB (3 mg.)
minimizes muscle
damage during
training and
increases upper
body strength.*
(Nutritional
supplementation of
the leucine metabolite
beta-hydroxy-beta-
methylbutyrate
(HMB) during
resistance training,
2000, Panton).

Strength Training Supplements
Which Supplements Really Work?

Advertisements for supplements that promote muscle growth and fat loss to be used with resistance training seem to be everywhere. Many supplements are effective in promoting muscle growth, and their benefits are proven by scientific research.

SHOULD SUPPLEMENTS BE TAKEN BEFORE OR AFTER TRAINING? A study at the University of Tennessee shows that protein supplements before *and* after training are helpful in promoting growth-oriented hormones during exercise and recovery (*Dietary supplements and promotion of muscle growth with resistance exercise*, 1999, Kreider).

Significant findings from this study:
· Chromium and vanadyl do not affect muscle growth, as once thought.
· Glutamine, creatine, and calcium beta-HMB have positive outcomes.

PROTEIN SUPPLEMENTS, before and after, but especially after training, promote muscle toning and growth.

Be careful to read more than the headlines about protein and other supplements. Recently, headlines read, "Medical Group Warns Against High-Protein Diets." This almost sounds like physicians are against protein in your diet.

Actually, the article was concerning research by the American Heart Association that shows that high-protein diets consisting of protein and high fat caused health problems because of the excess fat, not because of the high protein.

HMB (beta-hydroxy-beta-methylbutyrate) has been shown by researchers to increase lean body mass in several recent studies (*Over-the-counter supplements and strength training*, 2000, Joyner).

*"Strength
conditioning will
result in an
increase in muscle
size and this
increase in size is
largely the result
of increased
contractile
proteins."* (2002,
Effects of exercise on
senescent muscle.,
Clin Orthop,
Evans WJ.

CREATINE SUPPLEMENTS - Researchers conclude in a 2003 study that creatine, an amino acid, does not negatively impact exercise-induced growth hormone, and it may be helpful during strength training. Researchers report, "Creatine supplementation appears to be effective for maintaining muscular performance during the initial phase of high-volume resistance training..."(The effects of creatine supplementation on muscular performance and body composition responses to short-term resistance training overreaching, 2003, Voleck).

In a recent 2004 study, researchers report the latest findings on sports enhancing supplements, and the findings conclude that creatine seems to be safe. And creatine supplements do help with some sports that have repeated sprint performance involved. Creatine doesn't help, however, with a onetime maximal lift or a single sprinting event. Researchers report, "Creatine is ergogenic in repetitive anaerobic cycling sprints but not running or swimming" (Popular sports supplements and ergogenic aids, 2003, Juhn).

Essentially, creatine supplements help during a workout, especially at the end of a workout. And this is how creatine supplements ultimately improve performance. Using creatine supplements before workouts helps maintain intensity (more resistance, faster, etc.), throughout the workout, and this means enhanced muscle development, which, in turn, improves performance.

What about creatine for middle-age adults?

Personally, I've known many middle-age adults who have experimented with creatine supplements, and most of them gained around 5 to 10 pounds of water weight and, like me, ceased using the supplement. However, I have some very lean, middle-aged adult friends who have found creatine helpful when taken before training.

Researchers haven't settled on the issue of creatine for middle-age and older adults.

"Recent evidence suggests that creatine supplementation in conjunction with resistance training may elicit larger increases in muscle fiber cross-sectional area compared to training alone." (Nutritional supplementation and resistance training exercise: what is the evidence for enhanced skeletal muscle hypertrophy, 2000, Gibala).

"Most athletes ingest insufficient protein in their habitual diet." (Protein and amino acids for athletes, 2004, J Sports Sci , Tipton KD).

A 2003 study reports that 5 grams of creatine a day doesn't help. "It is concluded that long-term creatine intake (5 grams per day) in conjunction with exercise training does not beneficially impact physical fitness in men between 55 and 75 yr of age" (_Effects of creatine supplementation and exercise training on fitness in men 55-75 yr old._ J Appl Physiol. 2003, Eijnde EA).

Another research team reports that using 7 grams of creatine a day is positive. "Creatine supplementation may be a useful therapeutic strategy for older adults to attenuate loss in muscle strength and performance of functional living tasks" (_Creatine supplementation improves muscular performance in older men._ Med Sci Sports Exerc. 2002 Mar, Gotshalk LA). There will be more studies forthcoming as researchers advance science in this area.

ANDROSTENE was studied at length in 2000 at East Tennessee State University in the Andro Project. Androstene, made famous by baseball great Mark McGuire, caused a 16 percent testosterone increase after one month of treatment.

However, at the end of twelve weeks, testosterone levels dropped to pre-treatment levels. Why? The body's own production dropped to compensate for the initial artificial boost from the supplements.

Estrogen-related compounds (negative to muscle growth) increased along with other unfavorable cholesterol increases that, in turn, raised coronary heart disease risk. Neither strength nor body composition changed during the twelve-week experiment (_The Andro Project_, 2000, Broeder).

DHEA produced similar results to the Andro Project. During an eight-week study, DHEA did not increase testosterone, which is positive for muscle growth and the desired outcome of DHEA supplementation (_Effect of oral DHEA on serum testosterone and adaptations to resistance training in young men_, 1999, Brown).

New Research on Supplements

The GNC web site has information on supplements and drug interactions www.gnc.com. Detailed supplement information is available on an award-winning Web site produced by the U.S. Department of Agriculture www.nal.usda.gov/fnic/.

The National Institutes of Health have an Office of Dietary Supplements that is responsible for supporting supplement research and distributing research results, www.dietary-supplements.info.nih.gov.

For specific supplement, health, and fitness questions, the "Go Ask Alice" Web site produced by Columbia University www.goaskalice.columbia.edu/Cat3.html is an excellent source of information. This Web site provides a question and answer format to address specific issues, including questions that are generally asked confidentially.

The latest from researchers on dietary supplements:

Special sports foods, including energy bars and sports drinks, have a real role to play, and some protein supplements and meal replacements may also be useful in some circumstances. Where there is a demonstrated deficiency of an essential nutrient, an increased intake from food or from supplementation may help, but many athletes ignore the need for caution in supplement use and take supplements in doses that are not necessary or may even be harmful. Some supplements do offer the prospect of improved performance; these include creatine, caffeine, bicarbonate and, perhaps, a very few others. There is no evidence that prohormones such as androstenedione are effective in enhancing muscle mass or strength, and these prohormones may result in negative health consequences. (2004, Dietary supplements. J Sports Sci., Maughan RJ).

"We conclude that early intake of an oral protein supplement after resistance training is important for the development of hypertrophy (growth) *in skeletal muscle of elderly men in response to resistance training,"* (2001 Aug, *Timing of postexercise protein intake is important for muscle hypertrophy with resistance training in elderly humans,* J Physiol, Esmarck B).

"In addition to aerobic exercise, people should engage in resistance training and flexibility exercises."
(The evolution of physical activity recommendations: how much is enough? Am J Clin Nutr. 2004 May, Blair).

Stretch During Strength Training

Stretching during strength training is an absolute must if you want the full benefits of this program.

The 10-Minute Stretching Routine targets the lower body, and you can save time by stretching the upper body during weight training.

While working chest, for example, take 30 seconds between one of the sets and perform the javelin chest stretch on one side. Do another weightlifting set, then stretch the other side. The upper-body stretching positions are shown in Chapter 6.

Stretch the body part being worked is the rule for stretching the upper body during strength training.

Slowly move into the fully stretched position. Once fully stretched, you will feel the limit and the slight discomfort. Hold it for 30 seconds. Then, slowly ease out of the position. There should be no bouncing in order to reduce risk of injury.

In recent years, bodybuilders have begun to add stretching to their weight training.

Tactical Weight Training

The purpose of this section is to illustrate various strength-training exercises that target main body parts; chest, back, shoulder, biceps, triceps, quads, hamstrings, calves, abs, and obliques.

Specific exercises targeting these key muscle groups are placed in all five levels of Strategic Fitness Plans.

Individual body parts serve as the overall Target Zone for these exercises. But remember that you should also **zone-in** on the slow-twitch, fast-twitch (IIa), and the super fast (IIx) muscle fiber within each muscle group. This method will work all of your muscles, ligaments, and joints - and help you get the most benefit from your weight training.

Primary Exercises

Primary exercises are the proven weight-training exercises. They work major muscle groups with one or two main exercises. **Primary exercises are the gold standard** of resistance-training exercises.

Primary exercises will remain in weight-training workouts through the initial eight-week training period and beyond. Exercises, such as bench press, shoulder press, and curls, will be a permanent fixture for all five fitness training levels.

As you progress in the program and become stronger and better conditioned, you will need to add more resistance (*more weight, sets and reps*) and additional exercises to keep the progress going forward. The additional exercises are called "finishing exercises."

With each muscle group, there are typically several exercise options to select within the finishing exercise group. Finishing exercises are discussed on the following page.

"There is compelling evidence that prevention of weight regain in formerly obese individuals requires 60-90 minutes of moderate intensity activity or lesser amounts of vigorous intensity activity." (How much physical activity is enough to prevent unhealthy weight gain? Outcome of the IASO 1st Stock Conference and consensus statement. Obes Rev. 2003 May, Saris WH).

Finishing Exercises

Finishing exercises are used to **finish off a body part** after the primary exercises have been performed. Finishing exercises typically target a specific area within a major body part. Decline press, for example, specifically targets the lower chest.

Finishing exercises are in addition to, and always follow, primary exercises. Here you have options. Finishing exercises may be substituted with other finishing exercises, and the selection based on your preference - as long as the substitution is made within the same body part.

Some finishing exercises fit better with others because they work the same area. Also, exercise substitutions are suggested in each *Body Part Exercise Key*. Example: decline press and dips both work the lower chest, so it's suggested that you alternate these two exercises and not do them during the same workout.

Many experienced personal trainers change exercise routines for their clients at different periods to increase muscle stimulation. Some finishing exercises require special equipment; however, alternatives are provided.

Rotating "Finishing Exercises" every two to four weeks is a wise fitness strategy

Body Part Exercise Keys

Body Part Exercise Keys are provided for training Target Zones (major body parts). Each body part *Exercise Key* lists Primary Exercises and Finishing Exercises.

To emphasize the strategy that you are to target and really work a specific area of your body, a Lightning Bolt is placed in the center of the *Body Part Exercise Keys*. This graphic also divides the Primary Exercises from the Finishing Exercises. Following every *Body Part Exercise Key* are the photo-illustrations and descriptions of all the exercises by body part.

Remember, do not simply go through the motion of an exercise. Think Target Zone Training! Zone-in on one body part and target all three types of muscle fiber within every muscle group.

Furthermore, work the body part with exercises using the three principles of weight training: Isolation, Exhaustion, and Aerobic Recovery. And use the advanced E-Lifts strategy on all push and press movements.

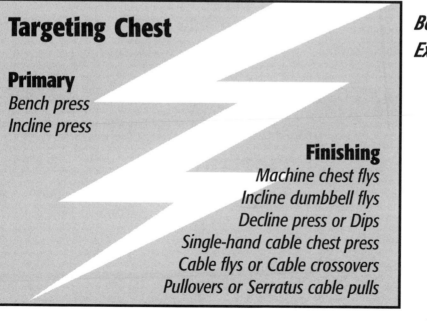

Targeting Chest

Body Part Exercise Key

Primary
Bench press
Incline press

Finishing
Machine chest flys
Incline dumbbell flys
Decline press or Dips
Single-hand cable chest press
Cable flys or Cable crossovers
Pullovers or Serratus cable pulls

Bench Press

Bench press is the weight lifting version of the push-up and it's excellent for **overall chest** development. There are many ways to perform this basic exercise that targets the chest muscles. The bench press is performed with a straight bar on a flat bench (with bar rack) as shown by personal trainer, Melanie Buchholz.

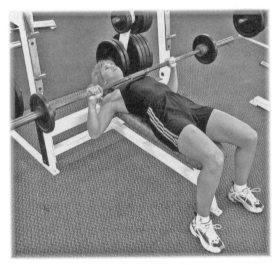 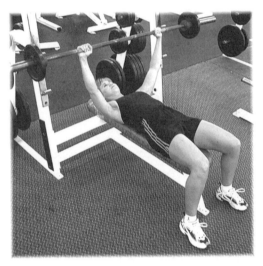

Lower position   Up position

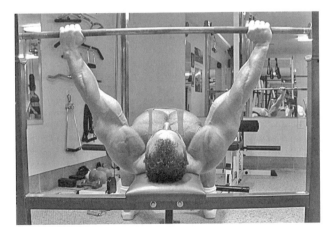

Nick Shelby, nationally ranked bodybuilder, demonstrates the technique of fully extending the arms between repetitions

Bench Press Alternatives

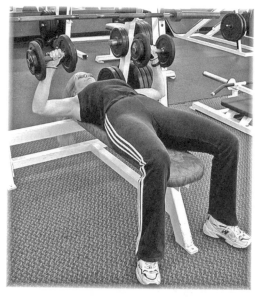

Dumbbell Chest Press

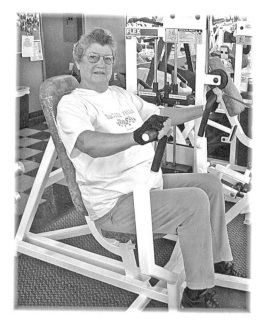

Machine chest press demonstrated by Pat Hutchison

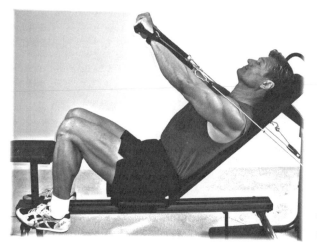

Incline cable chest press targets the upper chest. Cable exercises offer benefits to resistance training by adding variety and working muscles at different angles

Push-Ups: Great on the Road

The good old push-up is essentially a bench press with body weight resistance. It works the **chest** primarily. Push-ups are limited by having only one level of resistance - body weight. Free weights and resistance machines allow the selection of just the right amount of resistance, which will maximize results.

In a pinch while traveling, push-ups provide a good chest workout. Next time you are traveling, try the Hotel Room Push-up Routine. Do one push-up, stand, and tap a door facing once. Then do two push-ups, stand, and tap twice. Next, do three and repeat all the way to 10 (total 55 push-ups). I learned this workout from former professional football player, Dale Brady, 35 years ago.

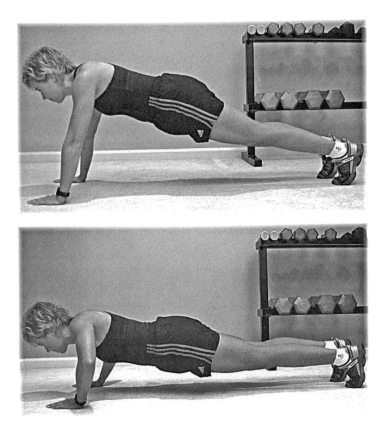

Incline Press

Incline press with a barbell is essentially a bench press on an incline bench with a bar or dumbbells. The incline shifts the focus of the exercise to target the **upper chest**. While more difficult than the bench press, this is my personal favorite for chest development.

Press up

Lower to touch chest

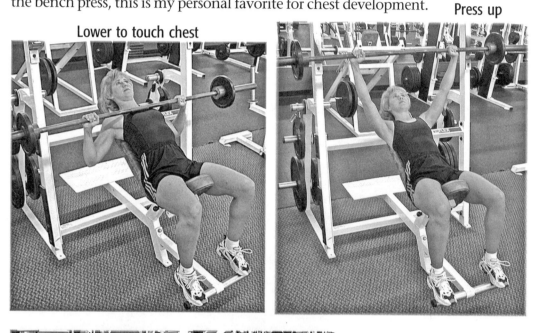

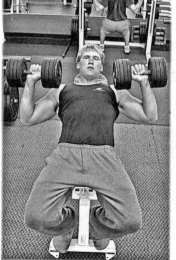
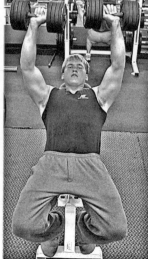

Incline dumbbell press demonstrated by Nick Friend

Cable Press

Cable chest press targets the **chest** similar to most chest press movements, however cable exercises offer added benefits to strength training by adding variety and working stabilization muscles and ligaments more than using a straight bar or dumbbells.

Cables, like dumbbells, require your muscles to work to stabilize and control the resistance (in every direction) in addition to the push movement of traditional weight training. Cable chest press engages the stabilizers even more than dumbbells, and this makes cable chest press a great finishing exercise.

There are great home gym units available that offer cable resistance exercises that target the stabilizers.

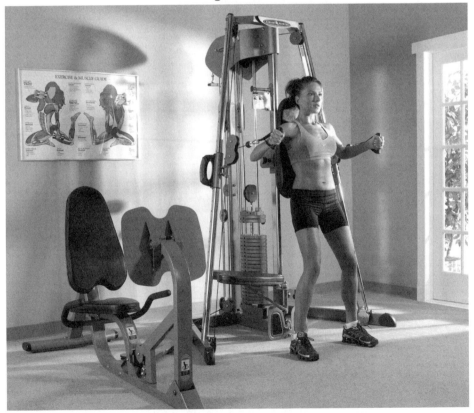

Functional Strength Trainer made by Vision Fitness
is available in most home fitness retail stores

Athletes that I train will generally perform three sets of cable chest press with E-Lifting tempo after first exhausting the muscles with several sets of Primary Exercises. They do three sets of bench and three sets of incline press as the Primary Exercises.

To finish off chest, the Finishing Exercises will generally be three sets of flys (standard tempo because this is not a push or press exercise) and three sets of cable chest press (shown below) with the explosive E-Lifting technique.

Strength Training at Home

Cable chest press can be performed standing or seated on advanced home strength training units. The new Functional Strength Trainer made by Vision Fitness is designed to handle the demands of explosive E-Lifting.

E-Lifts at home

Fitness Levels Two - Five should deploy the E-Lifts strength training strategy after warm up on bench, incline and decline press.

E-Lifts (*Chapter 9*) can be performed with free weights, commercial equipment available in most gyms, and at home. The home strength unit however, needs to be designed to handle the demands of explosive, high-intensity lifting.

Using independent, single-hand cables for a chest press exercise typically engages the stabilizer muscles. And this is perfect for many Finishing Exercises. However, it frequently takes more resistance on push and press exercises to exhaust large muscle groups.

The addition of a straight bar attachment (below) will resolve this issue by providing ways to perform Primary and Finishing exercises on the same unit. The straight bar provides more control so more effort can be placed into the explosive thrusting movement of pushing the resistance away from the body.

Cable stabilization exercises are perfect for newcomers. For the experienced and strength conditioned, single-hand cable Finishing Exercises are very beneficial when they follow Primary Exercises that have exhausted the targeted muscle group with E-Lifts.

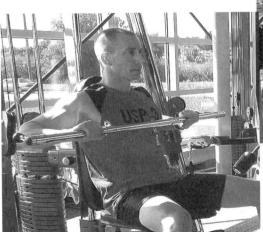
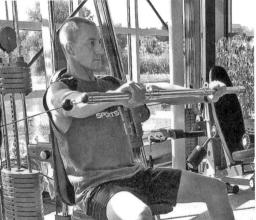

Cable chest press E-Lifting technique demonstrated by Dan Finn, Vision Fitness Strength Product Manager

Cable Chest Flys

Like all chest flys, cable flys target a specific area of the chest and serve well as a cable finishing exercise. What's the target area for flys? The rule: If the cable movement is below the chest (as shown below) the **lower chest** receives the focus. If the movement is above the shoulders, the upper chest is the target.

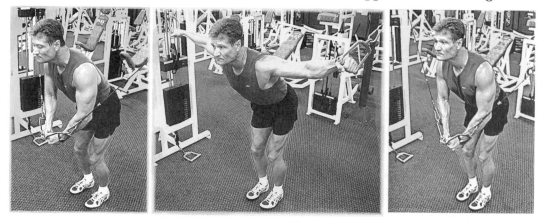

Start   Fly "out" position   Fly "in" position

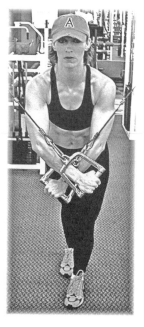

Cable Crossovers

Cable crossovers are similar to cable chest flys except the arms are bent more at the "out" position and the cables are crossed at the end of every repetition as shown by Shay Ingram.

Palms are faced toward your body during this exercise. Another version has the palms facing each other and this angle places the resistance on the lower chest.

Machine Flys

Machine flys provide a great workout. This angle targets the **lower chest**.

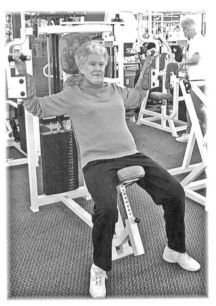

Decline Press

Decline press targets the **lower chest**. This exercise is the same as bench press but on a decline bench.

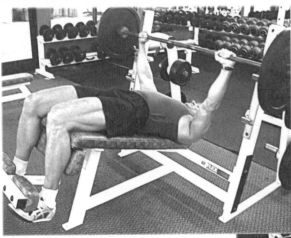

Joan Vidrine demonstrates machine flys.

Lower to touch chest

Start

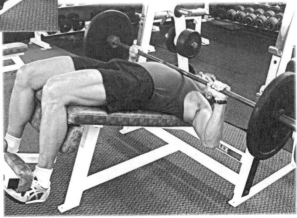

Dips

Dips work the **lower chest** and the triceps. Dips are similar to the decline press in their ability to target the lower chest. Use dips for chest development by going deep into the dip movement to stretch the chest fully. This is a chest finishing exercise that can be substituted within the chest finishing exercises listed in the *Body Part Exercise Key*, but it's best alternated with decline press.

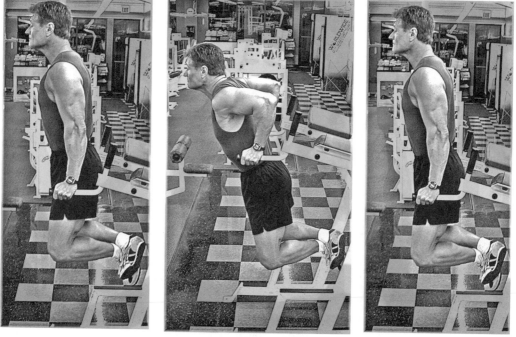

| Start | Deep dip position | Up |

Pullovers

Pullovers target the **ribcage area** of your chest. It generally only takes one set of 20 reps to work the ribcage area. This exercise also works the upper back.

Simply lay on a bench as shown, lower a moderate weight dumbbell back over your head until arms are parallel with the floor as shown. Fully stretch and expand your ribcage as you move into the out position.

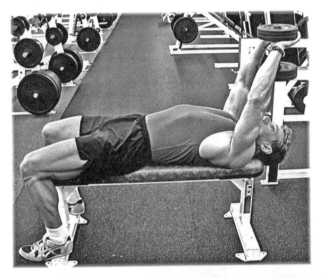

Out position - ribcage fully
stretched and extended

Up position
dumbbell is
over forehead

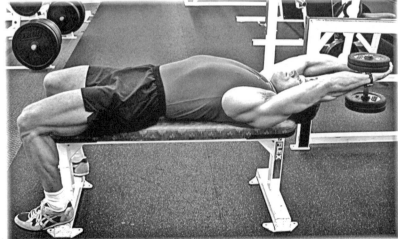

Serratus Cable Pulls

The serratus muscles are located just above the ribs, slightly below the chest (pectorals) muscles on both sides.

Pullovers work these muscles generally while the serratus cable pulls target these muscles directly. This exercise is somewhat difficult to perform correctly because hitting the correct areas takes some adjustment during the exercise.

This exercise is good for an occasional substitution for pullovers. The key is to focus on making the serratus muscles "feel the pull" of the weight. The repetition begins with a stretched straight arm as shown. Slightly pull down and in. Your hand should go down 6 to 10 inches.

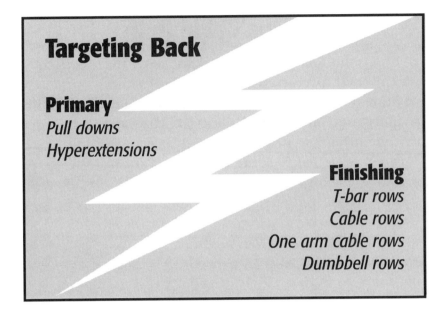

Targeting Back

Primary
Pull downs
Hyperextensions

Finishing
T-bar rows
Cable rows
One arm cable rows
Dumbbell rows

Pull Downs

Pull downs target the **upper back**. This exercise is performed by pulling the bar down, in-front of, or behind-the-neck.

The behind-the-neck movement isolates the upper back (lats). It's very important to make sure that you fully extend and really stretch at the top of this exercise while using the slower, traditional repetition tempo. Try and relax your biceps as much as possible and make your upper back does the work. And be careful not to bump your head; it's easy to do. I know from experience!

Some trainers teach clients to only pull the bar down in front. This may be a good idea for those training with very heavy weight.

The Ready, Set, Go! Fitness method of pull downs is to **work different angles** and make this two exercises in one.

Perform the first half of the reps behind-the-neck, and the last half in front *(as shown right)*. The upper-back muscles should fatigue during the behind-the-neck pull downs.

You maintain intensity by switching to front pull downs to finish the set. This method allows you to do more reps and fully exhaust the upper back muscles.

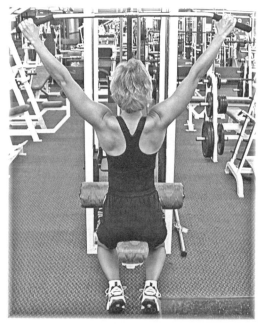

Stretch fully at the top of every rep

Pull Downs

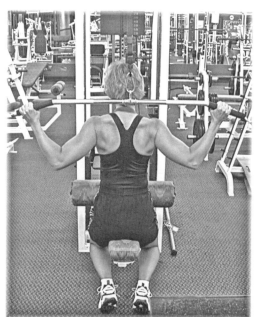

Pull down-behind neck

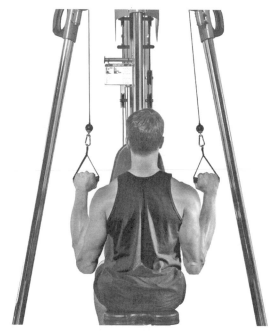

Pull Downs at home

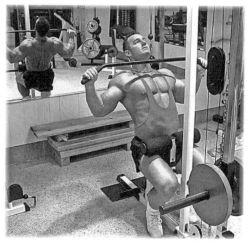

Front Pull Downs - Lean back slightly as the weight is pulled down

T-Bar Rows

T-bar rows are similar to other rowing exercises that target the **upper** & **mid back** areas. Start in a fully extended (stretched) position as shown, and pull the T-bar to the chest using your lats (upper-back muscles) to do the work. Careful - don't let your biceps do the work. Keep the focus on the lats.

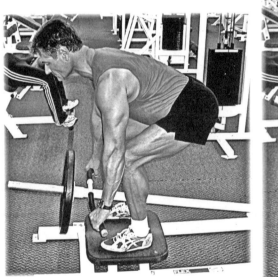

Start

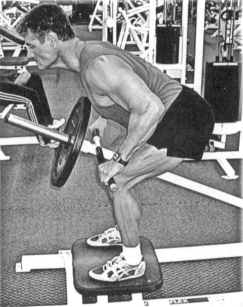

Up position

Cable Rows

Cable rows receive an A+ for their ability to work the **upper** & **mid back** areas. Start with your upper back straight, and fully stretched. Pull the cable toward your ribcage as shown. This exercise can also be performed with one arm for additional variation.

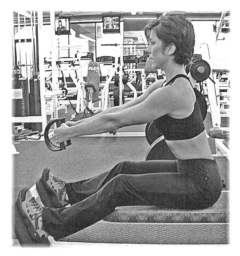

Start

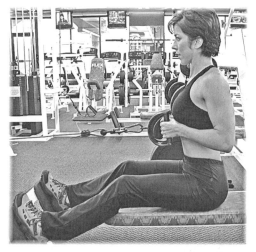

Pull back position

One Arm Cable Rows

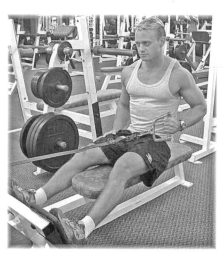

Kirk Pafford
demonstrates
one arm cable rows

Dumbbell Rows

Dumbbell rows target the **upper** & **mid back** areas and can be performed easily at home. As in all upper back exercises, fully stretch during the "down" or "out" arm position. And focus on not letting your biceps or forearms do the work. Correct body positioning is important to isolate upper back during this exercise.

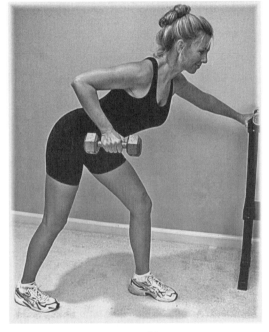

Up position

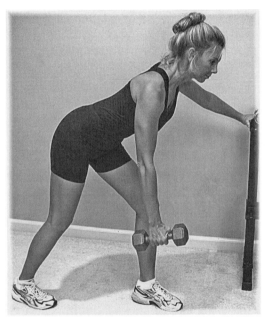

Arm extended down position

Hyperextensions

The **lower back** is the target area for hyperextensions. Go easy with this exercise and move slowly. I have injured my back with this exercise twice during my 37 years of weight training.

This is a great exercise for strengthening the lower back, but you must be careful not to perform it too quickly, or jerk your body through the movement.

Perform this exercise with hands on your chest as shown.

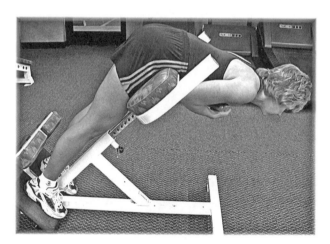

Lower position

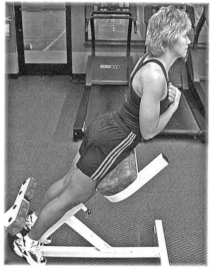

Up position

Targeting Shoulders

Primary
Shoulder press
Laterals raises
Shrugs

Finishing
Front raises
Rotator cuff rotations
Rear deltoid flys or Bent laterals

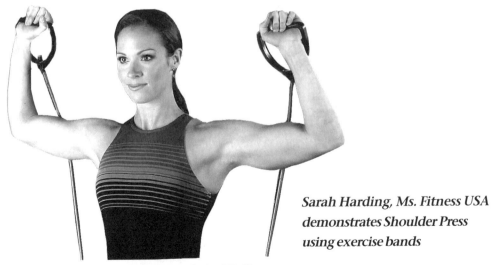

Sarah Harding, Ms. Fitness USA demonstrates Shoulder Press using exercise bands

Sarah Harding exercise photographs by TC Chang

Shoulder Press

Shoulder presses come in many fashions and are effective at developing the entire shoulder (deltoid) muscles.

Resistance training for shoulders can prevent injury, and also injure your shoulders if the training strategy is not on target. Kate Shelby, American Classic Fitness Champ, demonstrates the dumbbell shoulder press.

Having dumbbells at home can provide several high quality exercises to achieve a great workout. Note for newcomers and Fitness Level One participants: The "down" position for Level One should not come down below eye level. As you progress in the Levels, the more advanced technique of lowering the weight down to the shoulders may be used.

Down position

Press up position

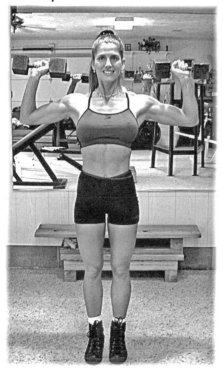
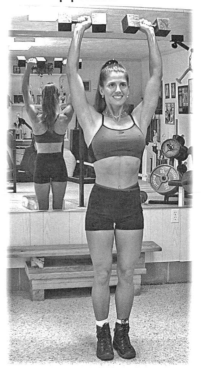

Shoulder Press

Seated barbell (*behind-the-neck*) shoulder press is an advanced exercise that isolates the shoulder muscles while reducing the stress in the lower back.

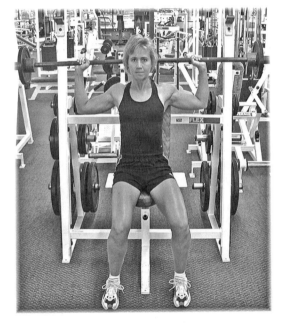

Lower bar to behind-the-neck

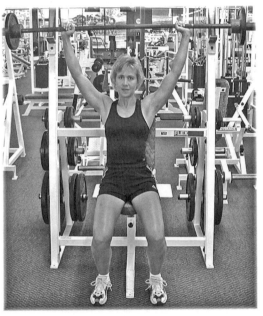

Press up position

The Ready, Set, Go! Fitness method of multi-tasking exercises to get better results and save time is performed by doing half the reps behind-the-neck. And the last half of the reps are done in front (*military press*) as shown *right* by nationally ranked bodybuilder, Nick Shelby.

Behind-the-neck weight training exercises tend to push the chest and shoulders forward and this positioning will stretch the shoulders, traps, and neck muscles more than lifting in front of the body. This exercise should be done with moderate weight and light weight for newcomers. Shoulder press with heavy weight should be performed in front, and not behind-the-neck.

Seated Shoulder Press is a variation that tends to support the lower back - especially for the advanced technique of lowering the weight to neck level.

This lower (neck level) position builds, but also stresses the shoulders. Even at advanced levels, before going below eye level with the weights, make sure your shoulders are warmed up.

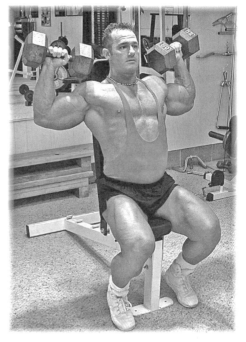

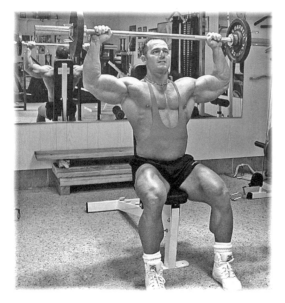

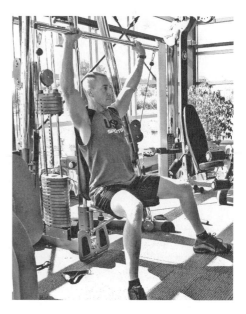

*E-Lifts at home
on cable
shoulder press*

Lateral Raises

Lateral raises target the outside center of the **deltoids** (shoulders). Raise the dumbbells from the side with straight wrists until you reach the up position (arms parallel to the floor) as shown.

Slightly bending the elbows as the dumbbells are raised will help isolate the deltoids and take pressure off the elbows. With high-intensity training, you should feel your shoulders "burning" on the last few reps.

Start with very light dumbbells until you get the feel for this exercise.

Start with palms in   Raise from the side

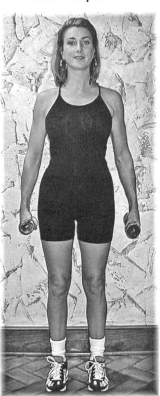 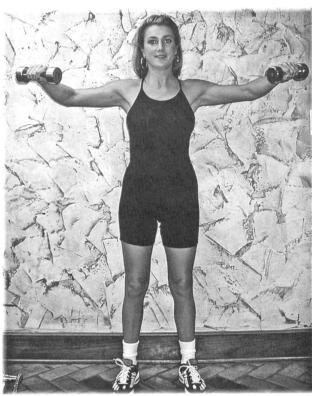

Lateral raises may be performed seated on a stability ball for additional development of torso stabilizing muscles, coordination, and balance.

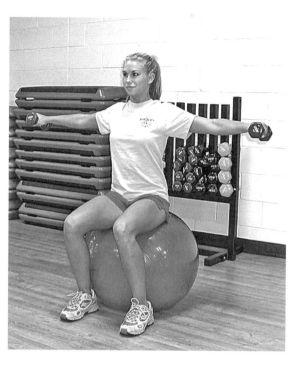

Laura Cole demonstrates lateral raises on a stability ball

Side Deltoid Twists is one variation to laterals raises that may be appropriate for someone needing to spend more time developing shoulder flexibility and strength.

Without any weight initially, hold the arms out to the side and stationary. Simply dip the hand forward as shown (like you are pouring water into a cup) then twist the hands backward. After you learn the movement, gradually introduce light dumbbells for resistance.

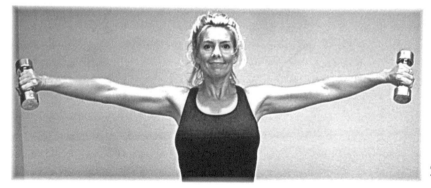

Side Deltoid Twist

Front Raises

Dumbbell Front raises target the **front deltoids.** Create synergy by multi-tasking this exercise. By keeping your palms down for the first 5–8 reps, and then finishing the set with palms-in on the last 5-8 reps - you'll be performing two exercises in one.

To reduce stress from the lower back, you should alternate arms and completely finish the rep with one arm before beginning with the other.

Keep your wrists straight and **slightly bend the elbows** to move the stress from the elbow joints and place the exercise target area on the front deltoids.

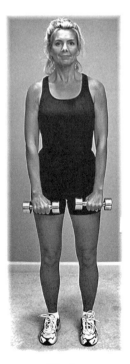

Start   Palms face down
               during first reps

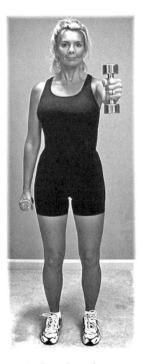

Palms face in
for last reps

Rotator Cuff Rotations

This exercise gets an A+ rating for effectiveness. **All ages should be performing this exercise** because if you live long enough, you'll likely experience rotator cuff problems. And this exercise will help to strengthen and protect this fragile area of the shoulder.

This exercise builds strength and flexibility in the injury prone rotator cuff area. This is a "must do" exercise for all women, and athletes that throw.

Using light weight, start with the weight at your ribcage as shown. **With elbow stationary and tucked** into your side, slowly rotate the weight to the outside, as far as possible, and return back to the "in position" before beginning the next repetition.

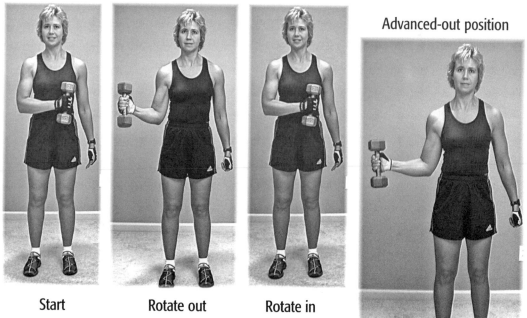

Start   Rotate out   Rotate in   Advanced-out position

Rear Deltoid Flys

Rear deltoid flys are typically performed on a Pec Deck or Chest Fly machine - except in reverse.

There are two ways to position your hands in order to multi-task exercises and work the rear deltoids from different angles. The Ready, Set, Go! Fitness method is to perform the first half of the set with *"palms in"* and the last half with *"palms out."* This method of multi-tasking fatigues the muscles quickly.

This exercise is the machine version of dumbbell bent lateral raises and it is somewhat similar to the swimming breast stroke. This exercise is a great finishing exercise for shoulders that will get the rear deltoids burning.

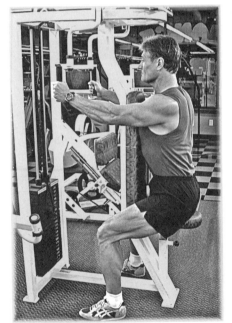

Start - palms in

Out position - palms in

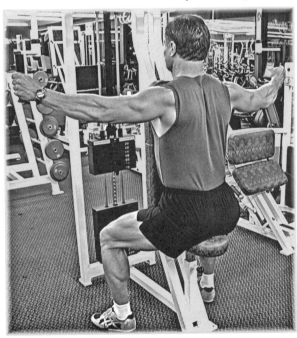

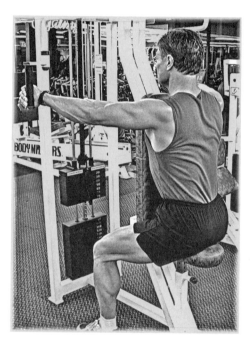

Last half of set
 - palms out

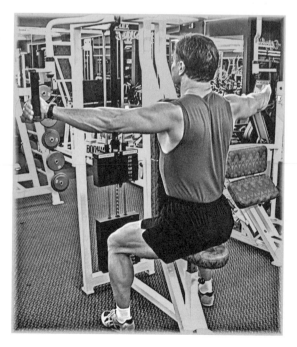

Bent Laterals

Bent laterals (or bent lateral raises) target the **rear deltoids**. This exercise strengthens the rear deltoid shoulder muscles, which are often neglected.

Start   Raise upward – palms down

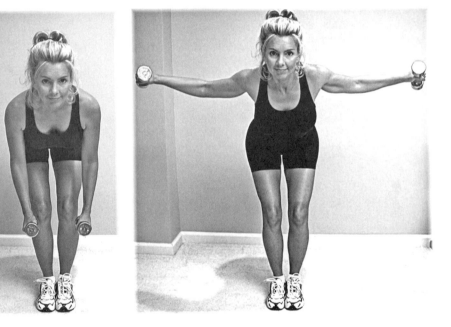

Shoulder Shrugs

Shoulders shrugs target the **traps.** Your traps (*trapezius*) cover a large area and runs from the top of your neck outward to your shoulders and about halfway down your upper back.

It's true that some football players want their traps to be so big that it frightens opponents. Shoulder shrugs, in moderation, will not develop your traps to this level, but shoulder shrugs will strengthen your traps.

Stress likes to zap the neck and the traps. Stress makes people tighten these muscles without realizing it. And the end result is head aches and neck tension. Shrugs will strengthen these stress-targeted muscles.

Rotate the shoulders up and around in a forward circle for the first 10 reps. Then reverse the circle for the last 10 reps.

Slightly bend the elbows and the knees during the circling motion.

When using heavy weight on shrugs, it's important to stay with the straight up-and-down motion, rather than the functional circular motion that may be used with light to moderate weights.

Start   Rotate shoulders – full in circle forward, then reverse

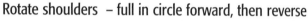

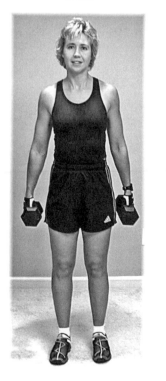
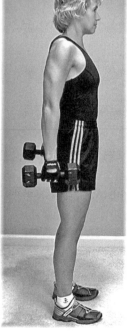
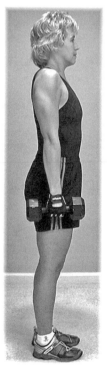
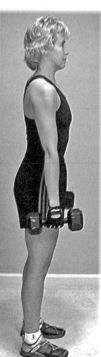

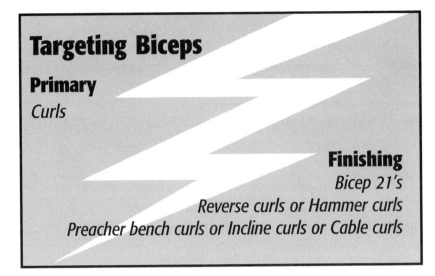

Bicep Curls

Bicep curls have taken many forms. And depending on the strategy, some methods are more effective than others.

Free weight standing barbell curls are the "standard." However, dumbbells provide a great workout and reduce stress on the lower back.

Barbell Curls

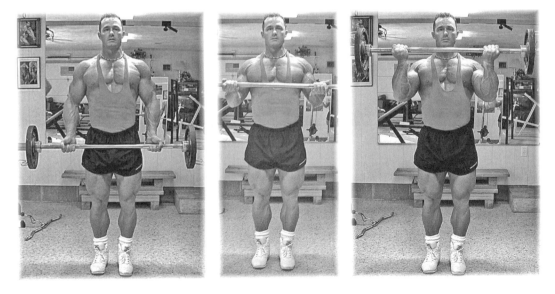

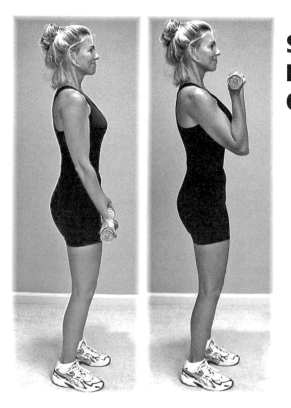

Standing Dumbbell Curls

Seated Dumbbell Curls

Seated dumbbell curls is a great exercise for all ages and fitness levels.

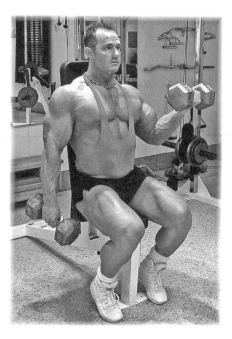

Incline Bench or Preacher Bench Curls

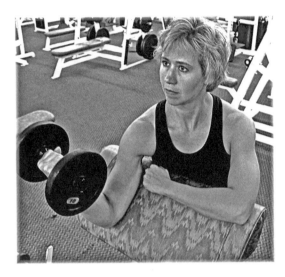

Preacher bench curls are performed with the arm positioned over an incline bench. This exercise inherited the name of preacher bench curls years ago.

Many machine curl units in gyms have an "incline preacher bench" feature that isolates the biceps.

Note: Always extend the arms fully on the down position.

Preacher Bench Dumbbell Curls

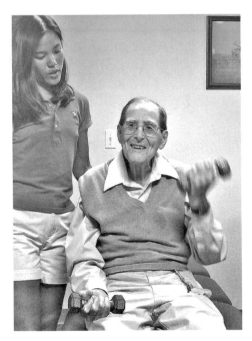

Max Riekes, age 97, demonstrates seated dumbbell curls with coaching from Paula Chan, MS, PT, ATC

Cable Curls at home on the Vision Fitness Functional Strength Trainer

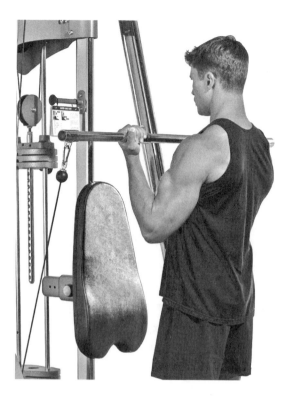

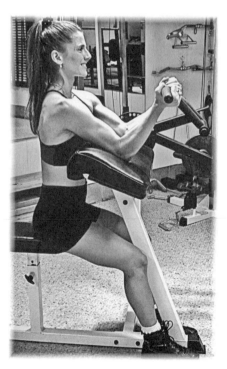

Machine Curls

Concentration Curls

Concentration curls requires focus to position your arm in a position to correctly isolate the bicep. Use your knee for supporting your arm as shown.

This exercise can be easily performed at home. Your knee may serve as the preacher's bench when one is not available.

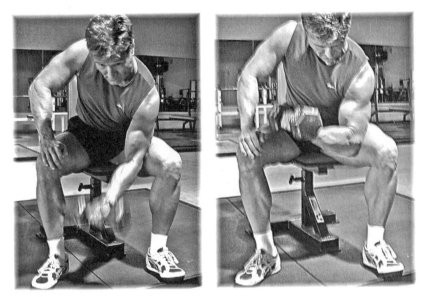

Curled position

Start

Bicep 21s

21s are my favorite bicep "finishing exercise." **Keep the dumbbells in your hands for 21 total repetitions.** First, do 7 reps from the fully extended start position to the halfway up position.

Follow immediately with 7 reps from the halfway point to all the way up position. Then do 7 complete reps for a total of 21 reps.

This exercise will achieve the desirable "burn" in your biceps. Bicep 21s can be performed on any of the curl exercises, however, the seated dumbbell curl and the concentration curl are well suited for 21s.

Hammer Curls

Hammer curls are always performed with dumbbells and alternating arms. This exercise targets both the **forearms** and biceps and is a great finishing exercise.

The curl is performed with palms facing in. The two main methods are demonstrated. The dumbbell may be raised up and straight out from the body as shown by Bambi LaFont, or may be kept close to the front of the body as shown by Nick Shelby.

Completely finish the rep with one arm before starting the next rep.

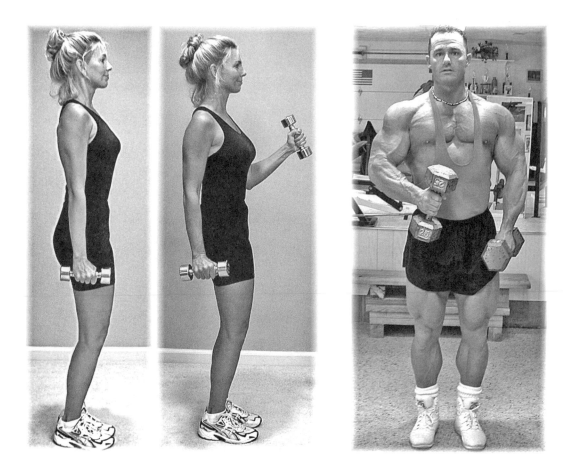

Exercise bands curls
demonstrated by
Sarah Harding, Ms. Fitness USA

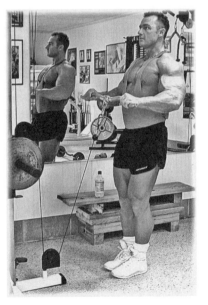

**Reverse
cable curls**

Reverse Forearm Curls

**Reverse
Dumbbell Curls**

Reverse curls move the target area of curls from the biceps to the **forearms.**

Reverse curls means that you simply reverse the curl palms up position to a *"palms down"* position as shown. Reverse curls may be performed with the barbell, dumbbells, or cables. Notice the "palms in" and "elbows tucked" to-the-side position.

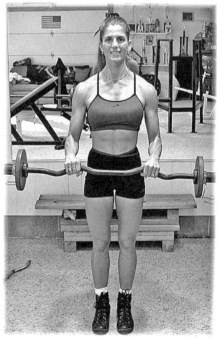

**Reverse Curls with
an EZ Curl Barbell**

Targeting Triceps

Primary
Press downs
Cable Tricep Extensions

Finishing
French presses
Tricep extensions or Kick backs
Reverse press downs or Reverse French presses

Press Downs

Tricep press downs rate an A+ for **targeting the triceps**. You can work triceps many different ways, but the press down gets great results for the entire tricep muscles (group of 3 muscles) if performed by the principles - isolation and exhaustion with aerobic tempo between sets.

There are two parts to Ready, Set, Go! Fitness Press Downs. On the first 10 reps, press the rope (or single handles) handle downward - with an E-Lifts outward flair at the end of the repetition (as shown right).

Once your triceps are exhausted (around 10 reps) and the flair out becomes difficult, begin pumping reps straight down - with the rope handle side-by-side (for the last 10 reps). This method should have your triceps "burning" by 20 reps.

The rope is preferred over the bar because it creates better isolation, and it takes stress off the elbow.

Personally, I find that it takes 20 reps with moderate weight to exhaust this naturally strong group of muscles.

Triceps tend to be a problem area for women. While "spot reducing" is controversial, extra work with triceps seems to have an impact on the triceps - whereas, waist spot reduction does not.

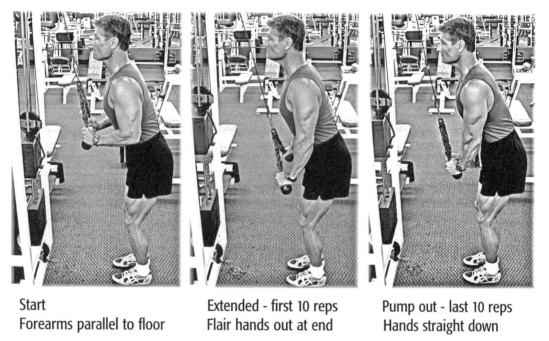

Start
Forearms parallel to floor

Extended - first 10 reps
Flair hands out at end

Pump out - last 10 reps
Hands straight down

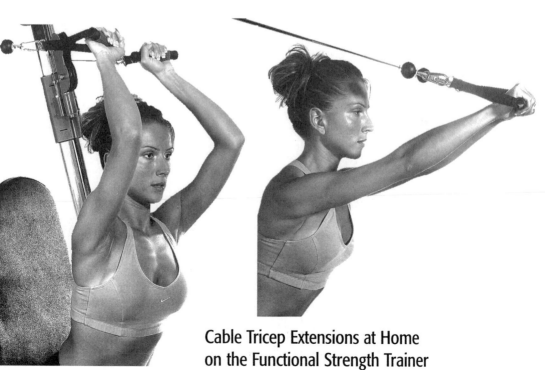

Cable Tricep Extensions at Home
on the Functional Strength Trainer

Reverse Press Downs

Reverse Press Downs is the same exercise as Press Downs, except the hands are turned upward as shown, and a bar is used rather than the rope.

This places emphasis on the outer part of the triceps. And this is a solid "finishing" exercise.

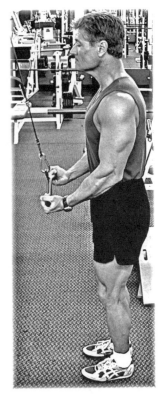

Start   Extended

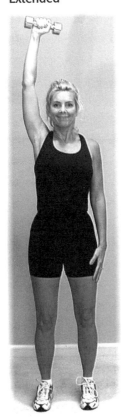

Hands
turned upward

Tricep Extensions

Overhead tricep extensions offer an excellent method for effectively working triceps. Warning; watch your head as you lower the dumbbell. Using a mirror to monitor your form with this exercise is recommended.

French Presses, Nose Breaks, Skull Crushers, and Hairlines... *all the same exercise*

Thirty five years ago, we called this exercise French Press. Today, the names vary, but the   results are the same. This exercise is a great tricep finishing exercise.

Careful with this exercise, it's definitely advanced. Why do you think someone named this exercise nose breaks, and skull crushers?

Hairlines might be a good name because you lower the weight to your forehead hairline and press upward while making your triceps do the work.

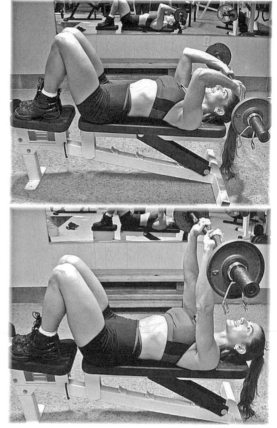

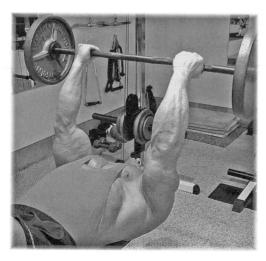

Reverse French presses. targets the outside head of the triceps.

Tricep Kickbacks

Tricep kickbacks rate an A+ as a tricep finishing exercise. This exercise is wonderful for women wanting extra work for their triceps.

Low weight and high reps will get the desirable high-intensity "burn" going.   And that is the goal with this exercise!

Want results fast: Make your triceps burn during resistance training. Careful, the tendency is to allow the shoulder to enter this exercise to assist burning triceps. Isolate the triceps by performing the exercise as shown, block the burning out-of-your-mind, and get great results!

Extended back

Start

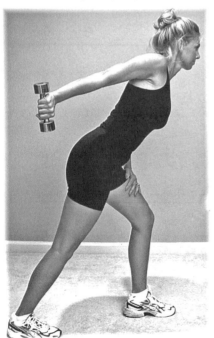
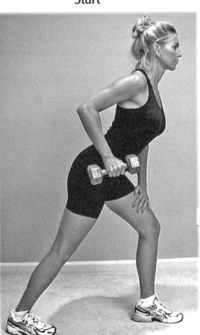

Targeting Quads

Primary
Leg press
Squats

Finishing
Leg extensions
Squat jumps
Hack squats or Front Squats
Dumbbell squats
Lunges or One-leg squats

Leg Extensions

Leg extensions target the **quads** (quadriceps), particularly muscles around the knees. Using moderate to heavy weight and sets with 20 repetitions will qualify as high-intensity work. Personally, I find that it takes 20 reps on leg extensions to achieve "exhaustion" during every set.

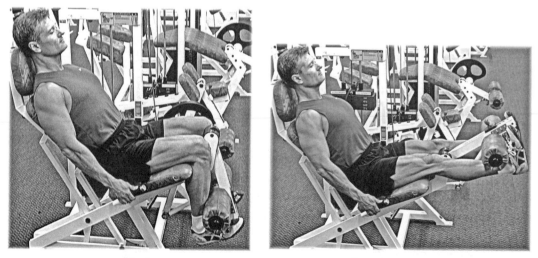

Start   Full extension, up position

Note - If you have ACL knee problems, checking with your physician may be a good idea before adding this exercise. **Protect your knees** - ACL thinning occurs in women over the age of forty. Should you experience any pain in your knees with any resistance exercise, STOP IMMEDIATELY, and see your physician. While ACL replacement surgery is available through advances in medical science to replace torn or shattered ACL's, surgery and months of rehab is not a good backup plan.

Squats

Squats score high as a muscle builder. Clearly, squats provide high-intensity training for overall leg development. Research from Duke University Medical Center shows that deep squats that go below parallel will increase the risk of injuring knee ligaments and the meniscus (*Knee biomechanics of the dynamic squat exercise*, Escamilla, 2001). **Don't go below parallel on squats!**

Start

Lower squat position

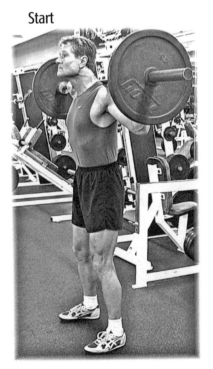
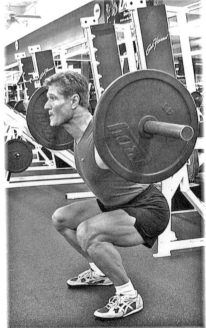

Thighs parallel to floor before standing.

Squat E-Lifts; pause for 2 counts in the lower position, then explode up

Speed-Strength Leg Training

One of the best workouts for speed-strength that I use with athletes preparing for the football Combines or Baseball Showcase events is squats or leg press (heavy weight with E-Lifts and reps in the range of 5 to 10) immediately followed by 10 reps of body weight squat jumps (3 sets).

There's no rest between the squats and squat jumps. The goal is to jump as high as possible on all 10 reps.

Using heavy loads during explosive resistance training may be the most effective strategy to achieve simultaneous improvements in muscle strength, power, and endurance in older adults. (Optimal load for increasing muscle power during explosive resistance training in older adults, 2005, J Gerontol A Biol Sci Med Sci. 2005 May;60(5):638-47, De Vos, NJ

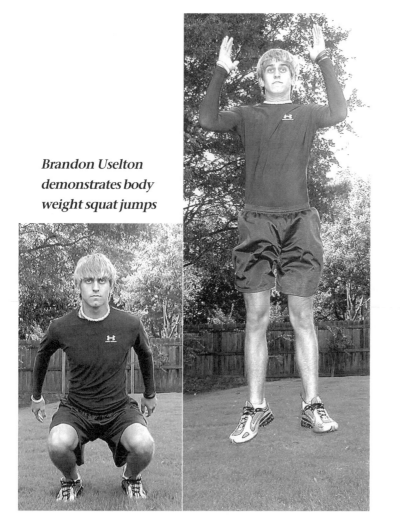

Brandon Uselton demonstrates body weight squat jumps

Front Squats

Front squats are a variation of the basic squat exercise. Front squats tend to isolate the center front part of the quads.

The best method is on the Smith Machine as shown. Thighs should be parallel to the floor in the squat position before returning up.

Start

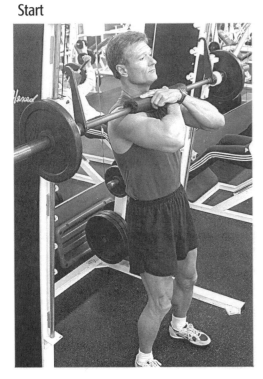

Squat position

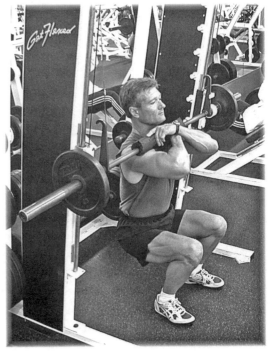

Dumbbell Squats

Dumbbell squats are easily performed at home, and perfect for Fitness Level One and newcomers to weight training.

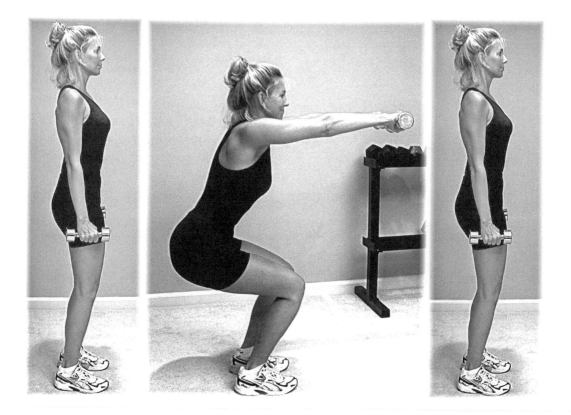

Leg Press

Leg press is a squat with back support. Leg Press, like squats, targets the **thighs** and the **upper hamstrings**.

This machine allows you to increase intensity by adding moderate to heavy weight. And your back is supported with this exercise.

Personally, I find that 20 reps with moderate weight produces great results. Need leg development? Try 20 reps on leg press. Keep the same weight that you're using now for 8 to 10 reps, and do 20 reps. Thighs are strong durable muscles that will respond to high reps with moderate weight.

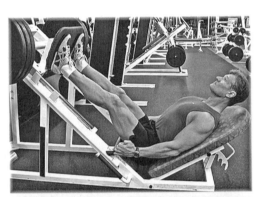

Up position

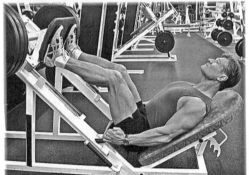

Midway position

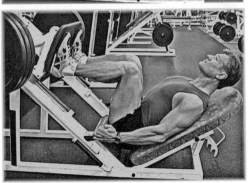

Down position

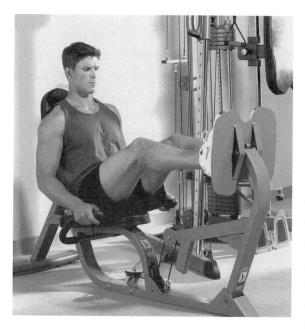

Leg Press at Home

Whether at home or in the gym, it's a good idea to add training variation in the form of single-limb exercises like the single-leg leg press demonstrated below by John Campbell.

Typically, if you're right-handed, the right side of your body will be dominant, and the left side will not be as strong. After working with thousands of athletes and individuals, I can say that this is almost universal, and it makes the case for adding single-limb exercises to your strength training program. The only problem is that it doubles the time because it takes two sets rather than one.

Researchers have also made the case that the lack of balance between legs, along with the strength imbalance between quads and hamstrings are responsible for many knee injuries in sports.

Essentially, the weaker knee is at risk because the strength is not great enough for the physical demand. And the dominant knee is at risk because the supporting muscles and ligaments are working too hard to compensate for the weaker side.

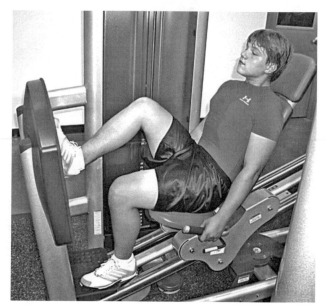

Lunges

Lunges are performed during plyometric workouts without weights (*Chapter 9*) and during weight training leg workouts - with dumbbells.

This exercise is great for your thighs, upper-hamstrings and gluts. Lunges can be performed easily at home. If you do not have a large room or a hallway to walk down during lunges, stationary lunges also work well. Stationary lunges can be performed by returning to the original start position after every repetition.

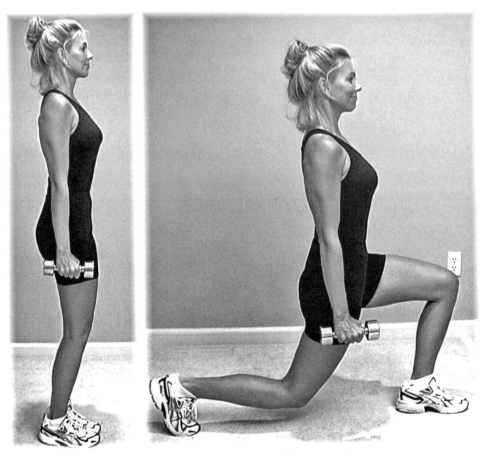

Start   Forward lunge position

One-Leg Squats

This is an advanced level exercise that is productive for developing quads and upper hamstrings, which are essential for sports speed development.

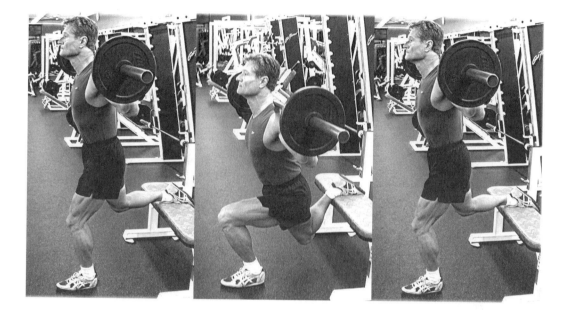

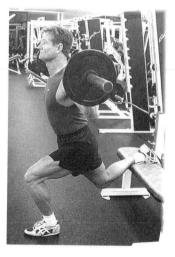

Until you get the feel for this advanced exercise, limit the depth of the lower position

Hack Squats

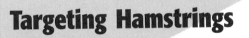

Hack Squats are a favorite for
developing quads. Hack squats
are essentially front squats with back support.
A wide stance with toes out works the inner thighs.
And a close, with toes straight, stance targets the
outer thighs.

Targeting Hamstrings

Primary
Leg curls
Single-leg curls

Finishing
Stiff-leg dead lifts

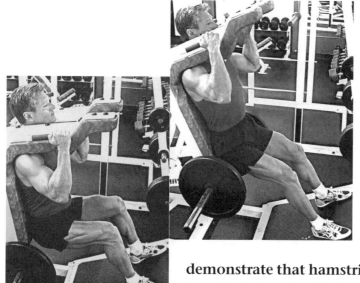

Hamstring strength and flexibility are important in many activities from sports speed development to injury prevention for the aging. Researchers in England demonstrate that hamstring strength and flexibility relate to low-back injury in active individuals. The researchers show that six months of hamstring strength training can contribute to a reduction in low-back injury (*Knee flexion to extension peak torque ratios and low-back injuries in highly active individuals*, 1997, Koutedakis).

Leg Curls

Hamstring development is generally lacking in most individuals and athletes.The balance between the quads (front) and the hamstrings (rear) always favors the quads. Typically, the quads are two times as strong as the hamstrings. And this ratio isn't desirable. To have the desired balance, the **hamstrings should be 75 to 80 percent as strong as the quads** (in a leg extension vs. leg curl test).

Want running speed? Want to improve athletic performance? Here is one key secret weapons; strengthen your hamstrings.

Experts report that most athletes have hamstrings that are 50 percent as strong as the quads (*Dintiman*, 1998). And this needs to be improved by 25 percent.

Improving the flexibility and strength of your hamstrings will do more than you can imagine to help improve performance. No matter what your age, college athlete or great grandmother, improving the strength and flexibility of your hamstrings will help you improve almost everything you do physically!

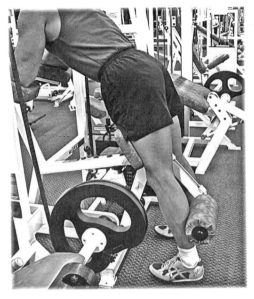

Start

Single-Leg Curls

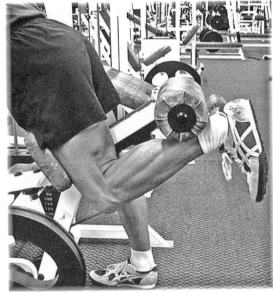

Curled
position

It's possible to work upper and lower hamstrings during the same set by changing the position of your foot. To target upper hamstrings during the first half of the reps, straighten your foot and point your toes away from the body (shown right).

Finish the set by targeting the lower hamstrings. Pull the toes up to a dorsiflexed foot position (shown above).

It takes concentration to straighten the foot during the first part of this exercise, but it should be very noticeable the area being worked when you change foot positions.

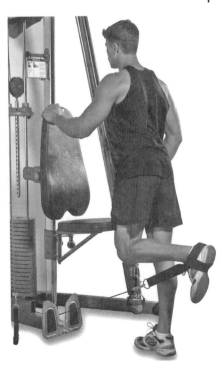

Leg Curls at home on the
Functional Strength Trainer

Dumbbell Leg Curls

Like the leg curls performed on the leg curl machine, a dumbbell and a bench at home provides a solid hamstring exercise. Holding the dumbbell with your feet makes the toes point and targets the upper hamstrings.

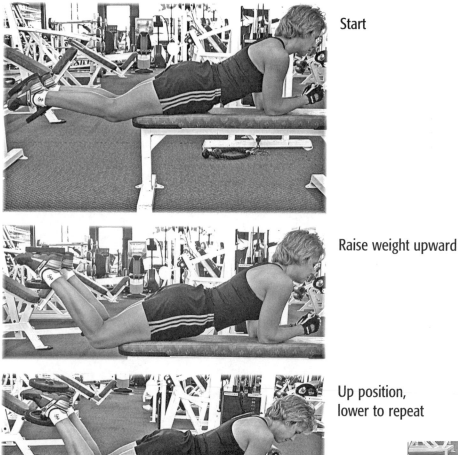

Start

Raise weight upward

Up position,
lower to repeat

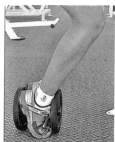

The trick to this exercise is placing the dumbbell between your feet (*right*) and carefully hanging your knees off the bench approximately 4 inches to begin the exercise.

Stiff Leg Dead Lifts

The lower back and upper hamstrings receive the greatest benefit from stiff leg dead lifts. Only don't keep your knees perfectly straight.

The name is "stiff leg," but slightly bend your knees and stop just past midway (as shown) until you are ready to move to more advanced levels.

Start

Forward- slightly bent knees

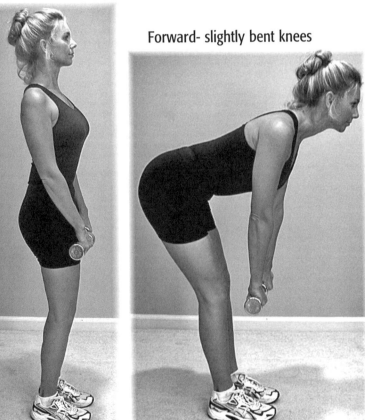

This position stretches hamstrings, significantly.

Since the upper part of the hamstrings is the typically the weakest point of your hamstrings, make sure you have been stretching for 60 days before performing this advanced position.

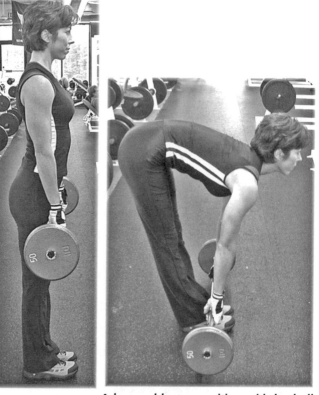

Kristi McCarver demonstrates advanced stiff-leg dead lifts

Advanced-lower position with barbell

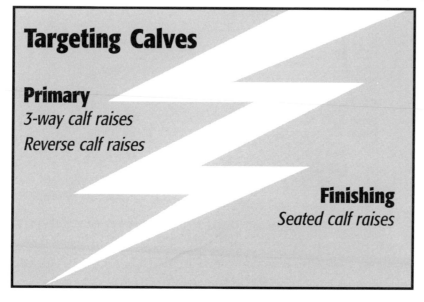

Targeting Calves

Primary
3-way calf raises
Reverse calf raises

Finishing
Seated calf raises

3-Way Calf Raises

Calf raises can be performed on a gym machine as shown or at home on a step.

Calves are durable muscles that take more reps to achieve exhaustion (20 reps per set).

The Ready, Set, Go! Fitness method targets all angles of your calves by performing the sets and reps in three different directions (*top right*). Example: If your Fitness Plan calls for 3 sets, then perform each set with your toes pointed in three different directions on different sets. If your Fitness Plan calls for 1 set of 21, then change positions every 7 reps.

Calf Raises at home
- just need a step

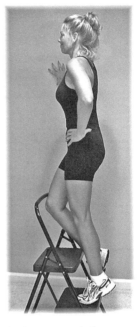

Fully stretch between reps

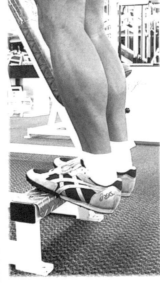

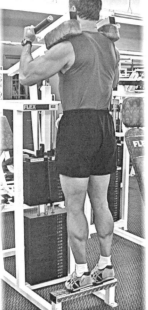

Gym
calf raise
machine

Important: To isolate calf muscles, it is essential to go down as far as possible and fully stretch your calves and Achilles tendons during every rep. Don't count the rep unless your heels go all the way down.

3-Way Calf Raises

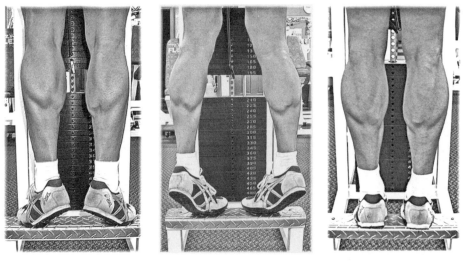

| Toes out | In | Straight |

Reverse Calf Raises

Placing your body weight on your heels and hanging both feet off the front of a step, positions you for reverse calf raises. Bend some at the hips (as shown), but keep your knees straight.

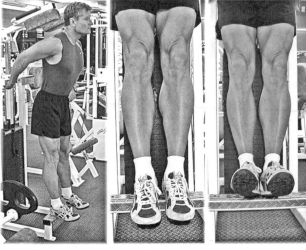

| Heals on step | Down | Up |

Seated Calf Raises

Seated calf raises work the calves in a slightly different angle than standing calf raises. This exercise serves well as a finishing exercise.

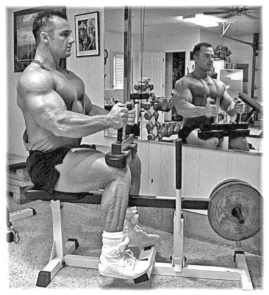

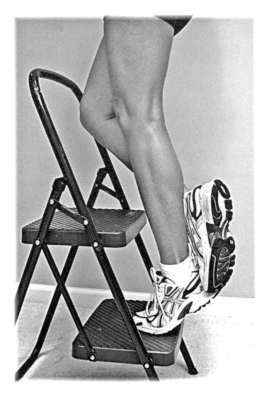

Calf Raises at Home

Calf raises can be performed with the resistance of your body weight - especially if you use one leg at a time as shown. All you need is a step.

Stubborn Calves?
Try the Sprint 8

The **Sprint 8** (*Chapter 8*) will develop calves, hamstrings and quads, unlike any other exercise I've seen.

If you have stubborn calf muscles, you may want to consider experimenting with working the fast-twitch fiber in your calves by sprinting and bleacher running to supplement weight training for calf and hamstring development.

Personally, I only do 3-way calf raises (3 sets of 20 reps) once a week along with the Sprint 8 Workouts (and no special dieting).

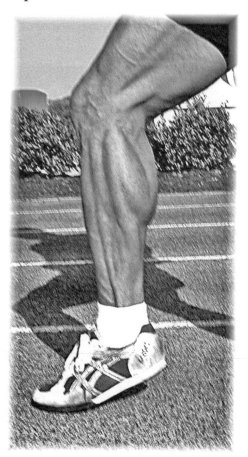

Traditional strength training primarily works slow-twitch muscle fiber. Calves are responsive when all three muscle-fiber types are worked (*Chapter 4*).

The *Target Zone Training* philosophy in this book suggests that you work your slow-twitch calf muscle fiber with traditional calf raises, and work your fast-twitch fiber with E-Lifts and with the Sprint 8.

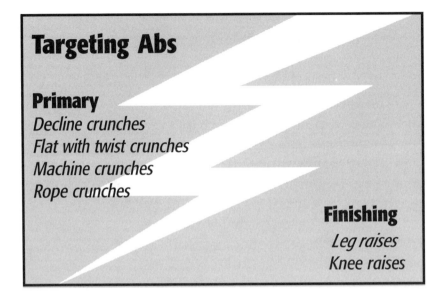

Targeting Abs

Primary
Decline crunches
Flat with twist crunches
Machine crunches
Rope crunches

Finishing
Leg raises
Knee raises

Decline Crunches

Crunches resemble quarter sit-ups and target the abs. Start in a fully expanded (ribs out) position, and roll your shoulders forward to crunch your abs. Keep your lower back touching the bench and raise your shoulders and upper back off the bench by approximately six inches.

Some call this exercise "cramp" sit-ups. This is a good description because this exercise sets your abs on fire. Decline bench crunches are great for adding intensity to the exercise.

Fully stretched, ribs out – start position

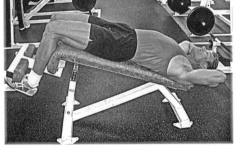

Up position

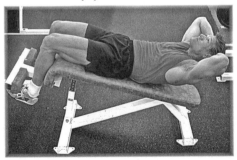

When you feel the "burning" in the abs that's the beginning of high-intensity training. The test is - how many reps you do after the burning starts. Personally, when the abs begin burning and I think I can't do any more, I quit thinking and try to block out the pain for 5 to 10 more reps.

It's a wise strategy to change the method of crunches every 30 days. Several alternate methods of ab crunches follow.

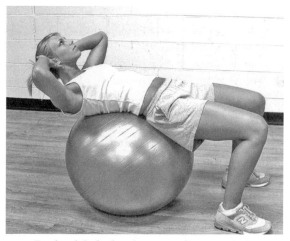

Rachael Cole develops coordination, balance and torso stability by performing crunches on a stability ball

Crunches

Crunches are sometimes called flat, mat, or floor crunches. This is a basic exercise for the **abs**. Crunches have replaced sit-ups because the sit-up places stress on the lower back - rather than working the abs. Crunches isolate the abs for high- intensity training and superior results.

Crunches - up position

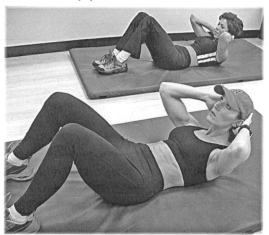

Crunches with twist

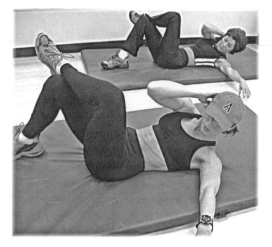

Machine Crunches

Machines for crunches are made by many strength training equipment manufacturers, and abdominal machines are usually available in most gyms. Today, some advanced home gyms offer ab crunch options.

While the ab machines seem to copy the basic floor crunch, some machines hit the abs in different ways making them a solid selection for crunches.

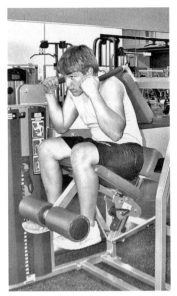

*Crunches at
Jackson Sport & Fitness*

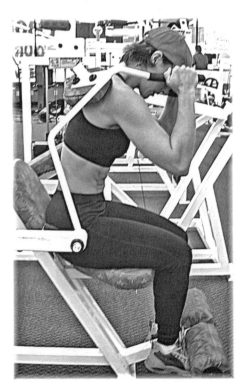

While conventional thinking is to use a high reps strategy for crunches, I prefer more resistance.

Torso strength is extremely important for many reasons and clearly, if you're going to perform high-intensity anaerobic exercise for a lifetime, you'll need a strong torso.

The thinking behind high reps for ab work originated back in the day when it was thought that "spot reduction" worked. Today, we know that it doesn't, so it's a wise strategy to build a strong torso by adding resistance to ab work.

Personally, I like enough resistance where 20 to 25 reps is difficult. When my abs start burning at 10 reps and I hang on for 20 to 25 reps, I've met the goal for the set.

Rope Crunches

Crunches, using a cable (with the rope handles), places high-intensity on the **abs** and some stress on the lower back. This is a great exercise, but use caution and monitor your lower back.

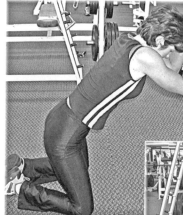

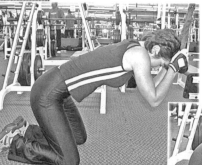

Pull toward floor

Fully crunched position

Start position;
rope in hands,
slight bend forward

Using the stability ball for crunches, as shown below on the Vision Fitness Home Functional Trainer, targets abs and the torso stabilizers while reducing lower-back stress.

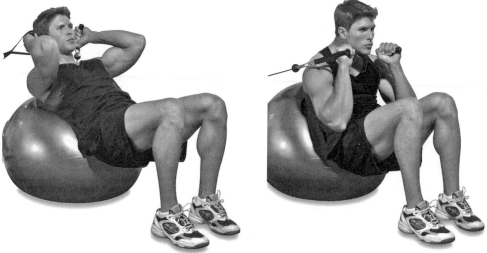

Leg Raises

Leg raises target the **lower abs** and hip flexors. Perform the flat, or floor, leg raises as shown.

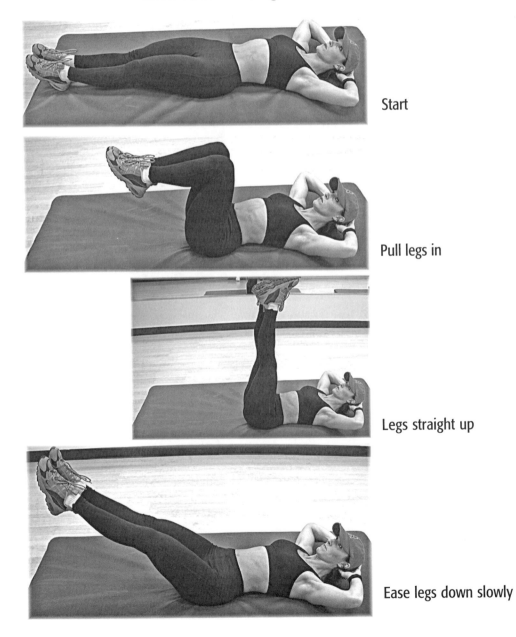

Start

Pull legs in

Legs straight up

Ease legs down slowly

Machine Leg Raises

Leg raises on the standing leg raise unit is a favorite for targeting the **abs** while reducing stress on the lower back.

The exercise is performed like the flat leg raises except you are leaning on the back of the unit (rather than the floor or a bench) in an upright, hanging position.

Start by raising your legs and bending the knees as shown, then lower them to the start position.

The advanced exercise calls for the legs to be straight. If you're somewhere in-between, perform the first reps with straight legs, then convert to bent legs for the final reps.

Start

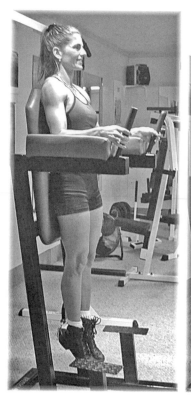

Raise - with bent knees

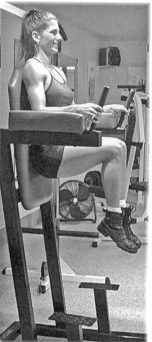

Advanced – legs straight

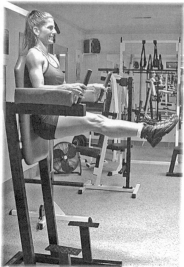

Seated Knee Raises

Seated knee raises offer a substitute for leg raises. Knee raises work the **lower abs** and may be done on the floor or a bench.

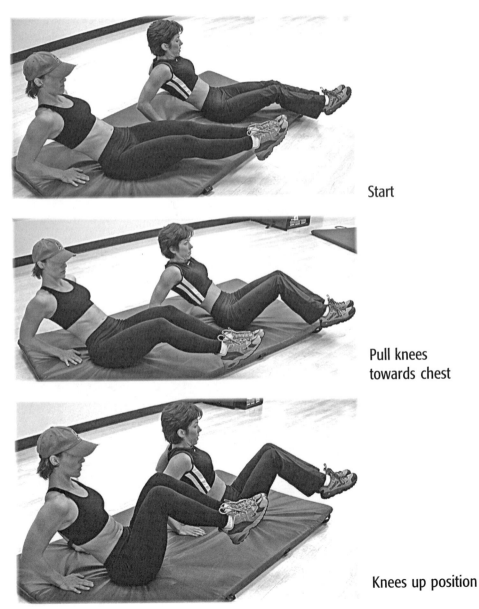

Start

Pull knees towards chest

Knees up position

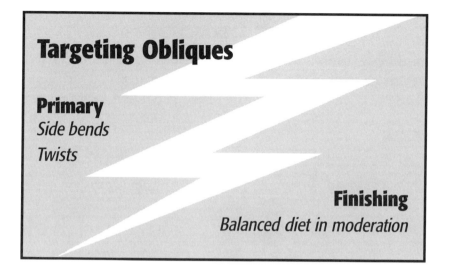

Targeting Obliques

Primary
Side bends

Twists

Finishing
Balanced diet in moderation

Side Bends

Side bends offer a quick and easy way to work obliques and increase flexibility in the lower back.

The all-time best developer of obliques is a balanced diet in moderation.

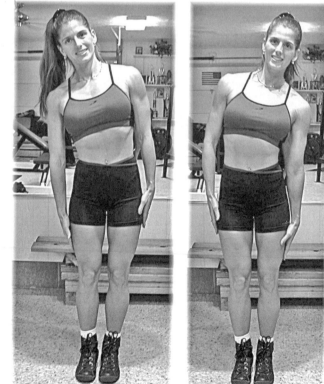

Twists

Twists seem simple, but this is a solid exercise for your obliques and lower back. This is a light exercise performed without weights because conventional thinking is that you do not want to use heavy resistance when twisting the lower back.

Arms up and twist from side to side

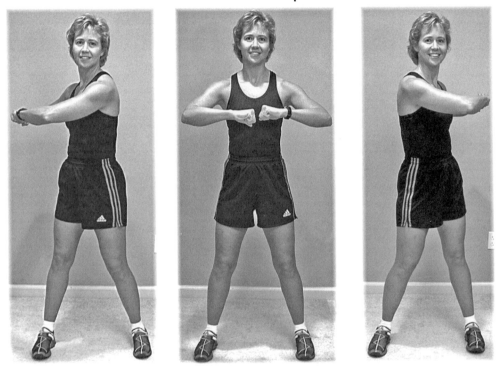

Throwing athletes that need a "whip" movement in their throws; baseball, football, softball, javelin, discus and shot, all live and die by the amount of "whip" they can generate in the throwing movement.

Essentially, a "whip" movement in a throw is generated by the athlete getting the hips and legs to the desired landing position quickly, while the shoulders and arms delay until the very last moment before the release of the throw.

The delay, and intentional separation of the hips from the upper body creates the "whip" (and twists the body at the waist). This means that the obliques, as well and as all the torso muscles, must be strong and very flexible.

When training athletes that throw in their sport for speed and strength, I use the Antwine Maneuver because I learned this technique from Orthopedic Surgeon and athlete, Dr. Trey Antwine.

In an effort to make the advanced version of Twists more closely resemble the "whip" in throwing movements, add a delay to the upper body (move the hips forward first), then follow with a fast twisting movement to the center by the upper body. The torso is in the middle of this movement and needs to be strong and flexible before using this advanced technique.

Typically, athletes performing the advanced version of Twists will use a straight bar on the shoulders and sit on a decline bench to increase the resistance on the obliques during the twisting movement.

Another variation of building the torso for sports specific movements, is baseball resisted swings (side woodchopper exercise) shown below by Dan Finn on the Vision Fitness Functional Strength Trainer. The handle rotates in the hands so baseball athletes and golfers can strengthen muscles specifically for the movements of their sport.

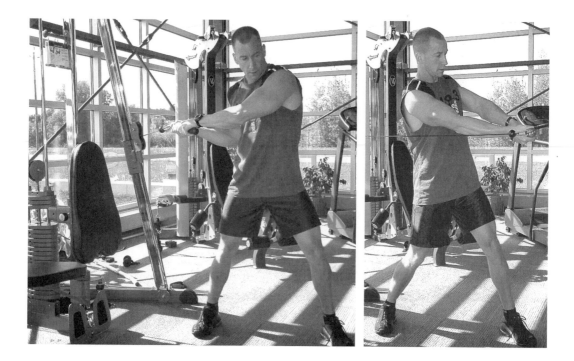

Conclusion

You have successfully completed the "Set" phase and now it's time to begin the "GO" phase by implementing one of the Strategic Fitness Plans in the next chapter.

All exercises listed in the Strategic Fitness Plans have been illustrated, and major components of *Ready, Set, Go! Synergy Fitness* have been discussed. Your Strategic Fitness Plan comes together in the following chapter.

Your book is a bible of health and fitness knowledge, thank you for taking the time to write it. You did an excellent job on format/layout of the book and the large lettering lets me read with ease while on the treadmill or bike. Thanks.
- Becky Collman, spin instructor

I purchased a copy approximately a year ago, and it has really made a difference in my life. I now go to the YMCA five/six days a week, and by using the "sprint 8" approach along with weight training, I have lost 18 lbs plus I'm also developing muscle lost after 30 years of no exercise.
- Dr. Don Coffey

This program was recommended to me by someone I met at the gym and since I have started it I have convinced 6 other people to buy the book and get with the program that works. **- John Von Mann**

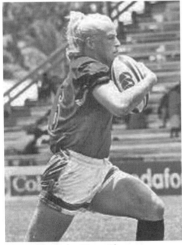

Photo by Steve Signes

Ready, Set, GO! is the tool I'm using to achieve my top levels of speed and fitness.
- Jen Sinkler, U.S. national women's rugby player

11

Strategic Fitness Plans

Ready, Set, GO!
It's time to start the GO phase!

Congratulations! You have successfully completed the **Ready** and **Set** sections, and now it's time to move into the action phase of Ready, Set, GO!

In the **Ready** section (*Chapters 1-4*), you learned how to increase exercise-induced hormone naturally and target your three muscle fiber types so you can synergize your metabolism, tone & build muscle, and turn your body into a fat-eating machine.

In the **Set** section (*Chapters 5–9*), you learned about the five major components of fitness training and how to correctly perform exercises that make up the Strategic Fitness Plans in this chapter.

Now, it's time to start the **GO** phase and begin receiving all the wonderful benefits of high-intensity fitness training.

Use This Chapter as a Workbook

Use this chapter as a workbook by charting the number of sets, reps, and weights used during training.

It's important to record notes concerning your training successes. By recording notes - during, and at the completion of your workout, you can track your fitness improvement and set training goals for the next workout.

Purchasers of this book may, for personal use, copy Strategic Fitness Plans in this chapter. If you don't want to write in the book, copies of the Fitness Plans are available at www.readysetgofitness.com/plans.shtml.

High-intensity fitness training is tough, and motivation to continue training will generally depend on seeing positive outcomes. Stick with your plan - daily and weekly - and you will see positive results.

Work the plan, and record your results. Research shows charting training results will yield greater success. The time you take to chart your progress will actually save you time.

Review Your Fitness Plan Before Every Workout

Before every workout, take 5 minutes to review your performance from the previous workout and think through the workout for the day.

Your Strategic Fitness Plan is designed to attack one day, and one week at a time. I can't overemphasize the importance of taking five minutes before every workout to review your plan for the day. This brief planning period will save you more time during the workout.

You are on your way to improved fitness, strength, appearance, and energy with every week of training. Use the proven planning principles - **plan your work, and then work your plan**. And remember to track your results. This will keep you focused and moving forward.

Fitness Training Levels

When in doubt, start with a lower Fitness Level;
you can always raise the Level at any point.

The five Fitness Levels are presented in Chapter 5, *Building Your Fitness Plan.* As you determine your starting training level, double-check which of the five Fitness Levels is right for you.

Carefully review the chart on page 106 and select the starting Fitness Level based on age, training experience, and current fitness status. This will insure that you begin with the correct Fitness Plan.

Level One is for newcomers to high-intensity training, adults over age 60, and children under age 14. Do not be misled; Level One is not a pushover program. It's demanding.

Level Two is for adults who have been exercising, but not with comprehensive training methods or with high-intensity workouts, and adults age 30 to 70. There is some overlapping with ages due to variables in fitness status at various ages.

Levels Three - Five are for physically fit individuals with fitness training experience.

These Levels include a split body routine for weight training (it is called "split body" because body parts are split and worked on different days).

As your fitness status improves, you will become more advanced in training. Remember, training intensity must increase to continue providing growth hormone release opportunities.

Exercise is a potent stimulator of growth hormone (GH) secretion. This study provides evidence that the GH response to acute exercise may increase lipolysis during recovery. Lipolysis is the breakdown of fat stored in fat cells. *(GH secretion in acute exercise may result in post-exercise lipolysis.* 2005 Oct 4, Growth Horm IGF Res. Wee J

Raising the Intensity Bar

With all aspects of Ready, Set, Go! Fitness; strength, flexibility, endurance, power, and anaerobic capacity, you will notice improvement quickly as you follow your Strategic Fitness Plan. To keep the results coming, keep pushing the intensity during each set and every workout.

Progressively bumping up intensity in your strength training means you will need to increase resistance gradually every few weeks by handling more weight, sets, and reps.

It may mean switching from a total body workout (Levels One and Two) to a split-body routine (Levels Three - Five) in a year or so.

Increasing the intensity level in flexibility means going just a little closer to the knee with your chest during the Hamstring Stretch.

Bumping up intensity in anaerobic sprinting typically means beginning with two to four sprints the first week and working up to eight repetitions by the fourth week.

After adding all eight sprints of the Sprint 8 Workout, intensity is increased by moving faster and harder, but not longer.

Increasing intensity may mean to pick up a a home cardio unit so you don't let bad weather interfere with your training schedule.

Measuring Performance of Your Fitness Plan

During your workout record the number of sets, reps, and weight used. Also make notes in the appropriate shaded boxes on the **Strategic Fitness Plan.**

Example: When you finish 20 minutes of cardio, write "Cardio-20" or "20 mins" in the shaded box under the day of the week that the workout is performed.

If you miss a day, use your ***make-up day*** on Wednesday to replace this workout.

Tracking your progress is critically important during the first eight-weeks of the program, but it remains important for continued success even after the initial eight-week period.

Training Logs for the first four weeks (for all five Fitness Levels) have been provided on the following pages. A sample of how a completed Fitness Plan should look after a few days of training is in Chapter 5, page 104.

Before you begin, go to the following Webpage http://www.readysetgofitness.com/plans.shtml and make copies of all four weeks. You will need these during the weeks following the initial training period.

Once the copies are made, begin recording results during your first workout - directly into the book or on your copies. And keep these records as a reminder of how far you have progressed.

STRATEGIC FITNESS PLAN
Level One

MONDAY	TUESDAY	WEDNESDAY	THURSDAY	FRIDAY	SATURDAY	SUNDAY
10-Minute Stretching Routine *Chapter 6*	**Weights** 30 minutes *Chapter 10*	**10-Minute Stretching Routine**	**Weights** 30 minutes	**10-Minute Stretching Routine**	**10-Minute Stretching Routine**	Rest
Sprint 8 20 minutes *Chapter 8*	**Cardio-20** 20 minutes *Chapter 7*	Make up day	**Cardio-20** 20 minutes	**Sprint 8**	**Cardio-20** or **Weights**	**TOTAL WEEK TIME:** 3 hours 20 mins
30 minutes	50 minutes	10 minutes	50 minutes	30 minutes	30 minutes	

Record your performance in the shaded areas

sample of completed plan on page 104

STRATEGIC FITNESS PLAN

Training Log   **Level One**   **Week 1**   **Date_____**

Workout:	Training Plan:		M	T	W	Th	F	Sat	S
10-Minute Stretching	**4 x week (M, W, F, Sat)** *Chapter 6*		▨				▨		
Cardio *Chapter 7*	**30 minutes 2 x week** *Tuesday, Thursday or Saturday*			▨					
Sprint 8 *Chapter 8*	**20 minutes 2 x week** *20-40% speed/intensity during first 4 weeks. 8 reps 70-yards, walk back.*		▨				▨		
Plyometrics *Chapter 9*	*Plyometric drills begin at Level Two*								
Weight Training:	**Exercise:** *Chapter 10*	**Record Sets & Reps** **Performance** *sets /reps*	*Record amount of weight used during sets in shaded areas.* **NOTE: Perform slow to moderate lifting tempo** *(up-on-two, down-on-four)*						
Chest	Bench press 1/12 Incline press 1/12 Chest stretch 30 sec	_____ _____	▨		▨		▨	▨	
Back	Pull downs 1/12 Up back stretch 30 sec	_____	▨		▨		▨	▨	
Shoulders	Shoulder press 1/10 Shrugs 1/15 Shoulder stretch 30 sec Rotator cuff 1/10	_____ _____ _____ _____	▨		▨		▨	▨	
Biceps	Curls 1/10 Incline DB curl 1/10	_____	▨		▨		▨	▨	
Triceps	Press downs 1/20		▨		▨		▨	▨	
Quads	Leg ext 1/20		▨		▨		▨	▨	
Hamstrings	Leg curls 1/12		▨		▨		▨	▨	
Calves	3-way calf raises 1/21		▨		▨		▨	▨	
Abs	Crunches 1/15		▨		▨		▨	▨	
Obliques	Twists 1/15		▨		▨		▨	▨	

STRATEGIC FITNESS PLAN

Training Log **Level One** **Week 2** **Date**_____

Workout:	Training Plan:		M	T	W	Th	F	Sat	S
10-Minute Stretching	**4 x week (M, W, F, Sat)** *Chapter 6*								
Cardio *Chapter 7*	**30 minutes 2 x week** *Tuesday, Thursday or Saturday*								
Sprint 8 *Chapter 8*	**20 minutes 2 x week** *20-40% speed/intensity* *during first 4 weeks. 8 reps 70-yards, walk back.*								
Plyometrics *Chapter 9*	*Plyometric drills* *begin at Level Two*								
Weight Training:	**Exercise:** *Chapter 10*	**Record Sets & Reps** ***Performance*** *sets /reps*	*Record amount of weight used during sets in shaded areas.* ***NOTE: Perform slow to moderate lifting tempo*** *(up-on-two, down-on-four)*						
Chest	Bench press 1/12 Incline press 1/12 Chest stretch 30 sec	_____ _____							
Back	Pull downs 1/12 Up back stretch 30 sec	_____							
Shoulders	Shoulder press 1/10 Shrugs 1/15 Shoulder stretch 30 sec Rotator cuff 1/10	_____ _____ _____							
Biceps	Curls 1/10 Incline DB curl 1/10	_____							
Triceps	Press downs 1/20								
Quads	Leg press 1/20								
Hamstrings	Leg curls 1/12								
Calves	3-way calf raises 1/21								
Abs	Crunches 1/15								
Obliques	Side bends 1/15								

STRATEGIC FITNESS PLAN

Training Log   Level One   Week 3   Date_____

Workout:	Training Plan:		M	T	W	Th	F	Sat	S
10-Minute Stretching	**4 x week (M, W, F, Sat)** *Chapter 6*		▓		▓		▓	▓	
Cardio *Chapter 7*	**30 minutes 2 x week** *Tuesday, Thursday or Saturday*			▓		▓			
Sprint 8 *Chapter 8*	**20 minutes 2 x week** *20-40% speed/intensity during first 4 weeks. 8 reps 70-yards, walk back.*		▓						
Plyometrics *Chapter 9*	***Plyometric drills begin at Level Two***								
Weight Training:	**Exercise:** *Chapter 10*	**Record Sets & Reps** *Performance* sets/reps	*Record amount of weight used during sets in shaded areas.* ***NOTE: Perform slow to moderate lifting tempo*** *(up-on-two, down-on-four)*						
Chest	Bench press 1/12 Incline press 1/12 Chest stretch 30 sec	_____ _____	▓		▓		▓	▓	
Back	Pull downs 1/12 Up back stretch 30 sec	_____							
Shoulders	Shoulder press 1/10 Shrugs 1/15 Shoulder stretch 30 sec Rotator cuff 1/10	_____ _____ _____							
Biceps	Curls 1/10 Incline DB curl 1/10	_____							
Triceps	Press downs 1/20								
Quads	Leg ext 1/20								
Hamstrings	Leg curls 1/12								
Calves	3-way calf raises 1/21								
Abs	Crunches 1/15								
Obliques	Twists 1/15								

STRATEGIC FITNESS PLAN

Training Log   **Level One**   **Week 4**   **Date**_____

Workout:	Training Plan:		M	Tu	W	Th	F	Sat	S
10-Minute Stretching	**4 x week (M, W, F, Sat)** *Chapter 6*		▨		▨		▨		
Cardio *Chapter 7*	**30 minutes 1 x week** *Tuesday, Thursday or Saturday*			▨					
Sprint 8 *Chapter 8*	**20 minutes 2 x week** *20-40% speed/intensity during first 4 weeks. 8 reps 70-yards, walk back.*		▨						
Plyometrics *Chapter 9*	*Plyometric drills begin at Level Two*								
Weight Training:	**Exercise:** *Chapter 10*	**Record Sets & Reps Performance** *sets/reps*	Record amount of weight used during sets in shaded areas. **NOTE: Perform slow to moderate lifting tempo** *(up-on-two, down-on-four)*						
Chest	Bench press 1/12 Incline press 1/12 Chest stretch 30 sec	_____ _____							
Back	Pull downs 1/12 Up back stretch 30 sec								
Shoulders	Shoulder press 1/10 Shrugs 1/15 Shoulder stretch 30 sec Rotator cuff 1/10	_____ _____							
Biceps	Curls 1/10 Incline DB curl 1/10	_____							
Triceps	Press downs 1/20								
Quads	Leg press 1/20								
Hamstrings	Leg curls 1/12								
Calves	3-way calf raises 1/21								
Abs	Crunches 1/15								
Obliques	Side bends 1/15								

NOTES:

STRATEGIC FITNESS PLAN
Level Two

MONDAY	TUESDAY	WEDNESDAY	THURSDAY	FRIDAY	SATURDAY	SUNDAY
10-Minute Stretching Routine *Chapter 6*	**Weights** 1 hour *Chapter 10*		**10-Minute Stretching Routine**	**10-Minute Stretching Routine**	**Weights** 1 hour	**Rest**
Sprint 8 20 minutes *Chapter 8*	**Cardio-20** 20 minutes *Chapter 7*	*Make up day*	**Weights** 1 hour	**Sprint 8**		
				Plyometrics *Chapter 9*		**TOTAL WEEK TIME:** 4 hours
30 minutes	1 hour 20 minutes		1 hour 10 minutes	45 minutes	1 hour	45 mins

STRATEGIC FITNESS PLAN

Training Log   **Level Two**   **Week 1**   **Date** _____

Workout:	Training Plan:		M	T	W	Th	F	Sat	S
10-Minute Stretching	**3 x week (M, Th, F)** *Chapter 6*		▨			▨	▨		
Cardio *Chapter 7*	**30 minutes 1 x week** *Tuesday or Thursday*			▨		▨			
Sprint 8 *Chapter 8*	**20 minutes 2 x week** *30-50% speed/intensity during first 4 weeks. 8 reps 70-yards, walk back.*		▨				▨		
Plyometrics *Chapter 9*	**15 minutes 1 x week** *1 set plyo-drills at half-speed*		▨						
Weight Training:	**Exercise:** *Chapter 10*	**Record Sets & Reps Performance** *sets/reps*	*Record amount of weight used during sets in shaded areas.* **NOTE: Perform E-Lifts** (Chp 9) on **push & press exercises**						
Chest	Bench press 2/12	_____							
	Incline press 1/12	_____							
	Chest stretch 30 sec								
Back	Pull downs 2/12	_____							
	Up back stretch 30 sec								
Shoulders	Shoulder press 2/10	_____							
	Front raises 1/10	_____							
	Shrugs 1/20	_____							
	Shoulder stretch 30 sec	_____							
	Rotator cuff 1/15								
Biceps	Curls 2/10	_____							
	Incline DB curl 1/10	_____							
Triceps	Press downs 3/20								
Quads	Leg press 2/20	_____							
	Leg ext 1/20								
Hamstrings	Leg curls 1/15								
Calves	3-way calf raises 1/21								
Abs	Leg raises 1/20	_____							
	Crunches 1/25								
Obliques	Twists 1/20								

STRATEGIC FITNESS PLAN

Training Log   **Level Two**   **Week 2**   **Date**_____

Workout:	Training Plan:		M	TU	W	TH	F	SAT	S
10-Minute Stretching	**3 x week (M, Th, F)** *Chapter 6*								
Cardio *Chapter 7*	**30 minutes 1 x week** *Tuesday or Thursday*								
Sprint 8 *Chapter 8*	**20 minutes 2 x week** *30-50% speed/intensity* *during first 4 weeks. 8 reps 70-yards*								
Plyometrics *Chapter 9*	**15 minutes 1 x week** *1 set plyo-drills at half-speed*								
Weight Training:	**Exercise:** *Chapter 10*	**Record Sets & Reps Performance** *sets/reps*	*Record amount of weight used during sets in shaded areas.* **NOTE: Perform E-Lifts** *(Chp 9)* on **push & press exercises**						
Chest	Bench press 2/12								
	Chest flys 1/12								
	Chest stretch 30 sec								
Back	Pull downs 2/12								
	Up back stretch 30 sec								
Shoulders	Shoulder press 2/10								
	Side raises 1/10								
	Shrugs 1/20								
	Shoulder stretch 30 sec								
Biceps	Curls 2/10								
	Bicep 21's 1/10								
Triceps	Press downs 2/20								
	Kick backs 1/12								
Quads	Hack squats 2/20								
	Leg ext 1/20								
Hamstrings	Leg curls 1/15								
Calves	3-way calf raises 1/21								
	Rev calf raises 1/20								
Abs	Crunches 2/25								
Obliques	Side bends 1/20								

STRATEGIC FITNESS PLAN

Training Log   **Level Two**   **Week 3**   **Date**_____

Workout:	Training Plan:		M	T	W	Th	F	Sat	S
10-Minute Stretching	**3 x week (M, Th, F)** *Chapter 6*		▓			▓	▓		
Cardio *Chapter 7*	**30 minutes 1 x week** *Tuesday or Thursday*				▓				
Sprint 8 *Chapter 8*	**20 minutes 2 x week** *30-50% speed/intensity during first 4 weeks. 8 reps 70-yards, walk back.*			▓			▓		
Plyometrics *Chapter 9*	**15 minutes 1 x week** *1 set plyo-drills*				▓				
Weight Training:	**Exercise:** *Chapter 10*	**Record Sets & Reps Performance** *sets/reps*	*Record amount of weight used during sets in shaded areas.* ***NOTE: Perform E-Lifts*** *(Chp 9) on* ***push & press exercises***						
Chest	Bench press 2/12	_____	▓		▓		▓	▓	
	Incline press 1/12	_____							
	Chest stretch 30 sec								
Back	Pull downs 2/12	_____	▓		▓		▓	▓	
	Up back stretch 30 sec								
Shoulders	Shoulder press 2/10	_____	▓		▓		▓	▓	
	Bent laterals 1/10	_____							
	Shrugs 1/20	_____							
	Shoulder stretch 30 sec	_____							
	Rotator cuff 1/15								
Biceps	Curls 2/10	_____	▓		▓		▓	▓	
	Incl DB curls 1/10	_____							
Triceps	Press downs 3/20		▓		▓		▓	▓	
Quads	Leg press 2/20	_____	▓		▓		▓	▓	
	Leg ext 1/20	_____							
Hamstrings	Leg curls 1/15	_____	▓		▓		▓	▓	
	Stiff leg dead lift 1/10								
Calves	3-way calf raises 1/21		▓		▓		▓	▓	
Abs	Leg raises 1/20	_____	▓		▓		▓	▓	
	Crunches 1/25								
Obliques	Twists 1/20		▓		▓		▓	▓	

STRATEGIC FITNESS PLAN

Training Log   Level Two   Week 4   Date_____

Workout:	Training Plan:		M	T	W	Th	F	Sat	S
10-Minute Stretching	**3 x week (M, Th, F)** *Chapter 6*								
Cardio *Chapter 7*	**30 minutes 1 x week** *Tuesday or Thursday*								
Sprint 8 *Chapter 8*	**20 minutes 2 x week** *30-50% speed/intensity during first 4 weeks. 8 reps 70 yards.*								
Plyometrics *Chapter 9*	**15 minutes 1 x week** *1 set plyo-drills*								
Weight Training:	**Exercise:** *Chapter 10*	**Record Sets & Reps Performance** *sets/reps*	*Record amount of weight used during sets in shaded areas.* ***NOTE: Perform E-Lifts (Chp 9) on push & press exercises***						
Chest	Bench press 2/12 Chest flys 1/12 Chest stretch 30 sec	_____ _____							
Back	Pull downs 2/12 Up back stretch 30 sec	_____							
Shoulders	Shoulder press 2/10 Side raises 1/10 Shrugs 1/20 Shoulder stretch 30 sec	_____ _____ _____							
Biceps	Curls 2/10 Hammer curls 1/10	_____							
Triceps	Press downs 2/20 Triceps ext 1/12	_____							
Quads	Hack squats 2/20 Leg ext 1/20	_____							
Hamstrings	Leg curls 1/15								
Calves	3-way calf raises 1/21 Rev calf raises 1/20	_____							
Abs	Crunches 2/25								
Obliques	Side bends 1/20								

NOTES:

NOTE: Continue the Fitness Plan for this Level until you complete your initial Eight-Week Commitment. For program continuation, additional copies of the Strategic Fitness Plans may be obtained from http://www.readysetgofitness.com/plans.shtml. All purchasers of this book have permission to copy plans for personal use. After the initial eight weeks of training, repeat the Fitness Level adding intensity (more weight, reps, speed), or move to the next Fitness Level.

STRATEGIC FITNESS PLAN
Level Three

MONDAY	TUESDAY	WEDNESDAY	THURSDAY	FRIDAY	SATURDAY	SUNDAY
10-Minute Stretching Routine *Chapter 6*	**Weights** 1 hour *Chapter 10*	**10-Minute Stretching Routine**	**10-Minute Stretching Routine**	**10-Minute Stretching Routine**	**Weights** 1 hour	Rest
Sprint 8 20 minutes *Chapter 8*	**Cardio-20** 20 minutes *Chapter 7*	*Make up day*	**Weights** 1 hour	**Sprint 8**	**Plyometrics** *Chapter 9*	
						TOTAL WEEK TIME:
30 minutes	1 hour 20 minutes	10 minutes	1 hour 10 minutes	30 minutes	1 hour 20 minutes	5 hours

STRATEGIC FITNESS PLAN

Training Log   **Level Three**   **Week 1**   **Date**_____

Workout:	Training Plan:		M	T	W	Th	F	Sat	S
10-Minute Stretching	**4 x week (M, W, Th, F)** *Chapter 6*		▨		▨	▨	▨		
Cardio *Chapter 7*	**30 minutes 1 x week** *Tuesday or Thursday*			▨					
Sprint 8 *Chapter 8*	**20 minutes 2 x week** *90-95% speed/intensity. 8 reps 70-yards*		▨				▨		
Plyometrics *Chapter 9*	**20 minutes 1 x week** *1 set plyo-drills*							▨	

Weight Training:	Exercise: *Chapter 10*		Record Sets & Reps Performance *sets/reps*	Record amount of weight used during sets in shaded areas. **NOTE: Perform E-Lifts** (Chp 9) on **push & press exercises**					
Chest	Bench press	3/12	_____		▨					
	Incline press	2/12	_____		▨					
	Cable flys	1/10	_____		▨					
	Chest stretch	30 sec	_____		▨					
	Pullovers	1/20	_____		▨					
Back	Pull downs	3/12	_____		▨					
	Cable rows	1/12	_____		▨					
	Up back stretch	30 sec	_____		▨					
	Hyper ext	1/20	_____		▨					
Shoulders	Shoulder press	3/10	_____				▨			
	Front raises	2/10	_____				▨			
	Shrugs	2/20	_____				▨			
	Shoulder stretch	30 sec	_____				▨			
	Rotator cuff	1/15	_____				▨			
Biceps	Curls	3/10	_____				▨			
	Incl DB curls	2/10	_____				▨			
Triceps	Press downs	3/20	_____				▨			
	Kick backs	1/20	_____				▨			
Quads	Leg press	3/20	_____						▨	
	Leg ext	2/20	_____						▨	
	Lunges	1/10	_____						▨	
Hamstrings	Leg curls	2/20	_____						▨	
Calves	3-way calf raises	3/30	_____						▨	
	Rev calf raises	1/40	_____						▨	
Abs	Leg raises	2/20	_____		▨		▨		▨	
	Crunches	1/25	_____		▨		▨		▨	
Obliques	Twists	1/20	_____		▨		▨		▨	

STRATEGIC FITNESS PLAN

Training Log   **Level Three**   **Week 2**   **Date**_____

Workout:	Training Plan:		M	T	W	Th	F	Sat	S
10-Minute Stretching	**4 x week (M, W, Th, F)** *Chapter 6*		▨		▨	▨	▨		
Cardio *Chapter 7*	**30 minutes 1 x week** *Tuesday or Thursday*			▨		▨			
Sprint 8 *Chapter 8*	**20 minutes 2 x week** *90-95% speed/intensity. 8 reps 70-yards*		▨				▨		
Plyometrics *Chapter 9*	**20 minutes 1 x week** *1 set plyo-drills*							▨	
Weight Training:	**Exercise:** *Chapter 10*	**Record Sets & Reps Performance** *sets/reps*	Record amount of weight used during sets in shaded areas. **NOTE: Perform E-Lifts** (Chp 9) on **push & press exercises**						

Weight Training:	Exercise:		Sets/Reps	M	T	W	Th	F	Sat	S
Chest	Bench press	3/12	_____		▨					
	Decline press	2/12	_____		▨					
	Cable flys	1/10	_____		▨					
	Chest stretch	30 sec	_____		▨					
	Pullovers	1/20	_____		▨					
Back	Pull downs	3/12	_____		▨					
	Cable rows	1/12	_____		▨					
	Up back stretch	30 sec	_____		▨					
	Hyper ext	1/20	_____		▨					
Shoulders	Shoulder press	3/10	_____				▨			
	Side raises	2/10	_____				▨			
	Shrugs	2/20	_____				▨			
	Shoulder stretch	30 sec	_____				▨			
	Rotator cuff	1/15	_____				▨			
Biceps	Curls	3/10	_____				▨			
	Bicep 21s	1/10	_____				▨			
Triceps	Press downs	3/20	_____				▨			
	French press	1/20	_____				▨			
Quads	Leg press	3/20	_____						▨	
	One-leg leg ext	2/20	_____						▨	
Hamstrings	Leg curls	2/20	_____						▨	
	Stiff dead lift	1/10	_____						▨	
Calves	3-way calf raises	3/30	_____						▨	
Abs	Leg raises	2/20	_____			▨	▨		▨	
	Crunches	1/25	_____			▨	▨		▨	
Obliques	Side bends	1/20	_____						▨	

STRATEGIC FITNESS PLAN

Training Log   Level Three   Week 3   Date_____

Workout:	Training Plan:	M	T	W	Th	F	Sat	S
10-Minute Stretching	**4 x week (M, W, Th, F)** *Chapter 6*	▨		▨	▨	▨		
Cardio *Chapter 7*	**30 minutes 1 x week** *Tuesday or Thursday*							
Sprint 8 *Chapter 8*	**20 minutes 2 x week** *90-95% speed/intensity. 8 reps 70-yards*	▨				▨		
Plyometrics *Chapter 9*	**20 minutes 1 x week** *1 set plyo-drills*						▨	

Weight Training:	Exercise: *Chapter 10*	Record Sets & Reps Performance *sets/reps*	Record amount of weight used during sets in shaded areas. **NOTE: Perform E-Lifts (Chp 9) on push & press exercises**					

Weight Training	Exercise	Record Sets & Reps Performance sets/reps	M	T	W	Th	F	Sat	S
Chest	Bench press 3/12 / Incline press 2/12 / Cable flys 1/10 / Chest stretch 30 sec / Pullovers 1/20	_____ _____ _____ _____ _____		▨					
Back	Pull downs 3/12 / T-bar rows 1/12 / Up back stretch 30 sec / Hyper ext 1/20	_____ _____ _____ _____		▨					
Shoulders	Shoulder press 3/10 / Front raises 2/10 / Shrugs 2/20 / Shoulder stretch 30 sec / Rotator cuff 1/15	_____ _____ _____ _____ _____				▨			
Biceps	Curls 3/10 / Incl DB curls 2/10 / Hammer curls 1/10	_____ _____ _____				▨			
Triceps	Press downs 3/20 / Rev press downs 1/20	_____ _____		▨					
Quads	Leg press 3/20 / Leg ext 2/20 / Lunges 1/10	_____ _____ _____						▨	
Hamstrings	Leg curls 2/20	_____						▨	
Calves	3-way calf raises 3/30 / Rev calf raises 1/40	_____ _____							
Abs	Leg raises 2/20 / Crunches 1/25	_____ _____		▨		▨			
Obliques	Twists 1/20								

STRATEGIC FITNESS PLAN

Training Log   **Level Three**   **Week 4**   **Date**_____

Workout:	Training Plan:		M	T	W	Th	F	Sat	S
10-Minute Stretching	**4 x week (M, W, Th, F)** *Chapter 6*		▓		▓	▓	▓		
Cardio *Chapter 7*	**30 minutes 1 x week** *Tuesday or Thursday*			▓					
Sprint 8 *Chapter 8*	**20 minutes 2 x week** *90-95% speed/intensity. 8 reps 70-yards*		▓			▓			
Plyometrics *Chapter 9*	**20 minutes 1 x week** *1 set plyo-drills*							▓	

Weight Training:	Exercise: *Chapter 10*	Record Sets & Reps Performance *sets/reps*	Record amount of weight used during sets in shaded areas. **NOTE: Perform E-Lifts** *(Chp 9)* on **push & press exercises**						
Chest	Bench press 3/12 Decline press 2/12 Cable flys 1/10 Chest stretch 30 sec Pullovers 1/20	▓		▓					
Back	Pull downs 3/12 Cable rows 1/12 Up back stretch 30 sec Hyper ext 1/20	▓		▓					
Shoulders	Shoulder press 3/10 Side raises 2/10 Shrugs 2/20 Shoulder stretch 30 sec Rotator cuff 1/15	▓				▓			
Biceps	Curls 3/10 Bicep 21s 1/10	▓				▓			
Triceps	Press downs 3/20 Tricep ext 1/20	▓				▓			
Quads	Leg press 3/20 One-leg leg ext 2/10	▓						▓	
Hamstrings	Leg curls 2/20 Stiff dead lift 1/10	▓						▓	
Calves	3-way calf raises 3/30	▓						▓	
Abs	Leg raises 2/20 Crunches 1/25	▓		▓		▓			
Obliques	Side bends 1/20	▓							

NOTES:

STRATEGIC FITNESS PLAN
Level Four

MONDAY	TUESDAY	WEDNESDAY	THURSDAY	FRIDAY	SATURDAY	SUNDAY
10-Minute Stretching Routine *Chapter 6*	**10-Minute Stretching Routine**		**10-Minute Stretching Routine**		**10-Minute Stretching Routine**	Rest
Sprint 8 20 minutes *Chapter 8*	**Plyometrics** 20 minutes *Chapter 9*	*Make up day*	**Sprint 8**	**Cardio-30** *Chapter 7*	**Sprint 8**	
Weights 1 hour *Chapter 10*	**Weights** 1 hour		**Weights** 1 hour		**Weights** 1 hour	
						TOTAL WEEK TIME:
1 hour 30 minutes	1 hour 30 minutes		1 hour 30 minutes	30 minutes	1 hour 30 minutes	6 hours 30 minutes

Before beginning Level Four, you should be experienced in sprinting, weightlifting, and the other components of *Ready, Set, Go! Fitness.*

Note for speed training athletes: If you are training for speed improvement and using Level Four or Level Five, your 10-Minute Stretching Routine should be performed after sprinting workouts so you will not impair sprinting performance during training.

Static stretching builds flexibility, however, it can slightly slow down your running speed for an hour after stretching, which is fine, and even desirable for individuals running the Sprint 8 for fitness improvement.

Athletes training for speed must *train fast to be fast,* so it's important to warm up before sprinting with a dynamic warm up like joint circles and plyometric drills, and perform the 10-Minute Stretching Routine after training.

STRATEGIC FITNESS PLAN

Training Log   Level Four   Week 1   Date_____

Workout:	Training Plan:		M	T	W	Th	F	Sat	S
10-Minute Stretching	**4 x week (M, T, Th, Sat)** *Chapter 6*		▓	▓		▓		▓	
Cardio *Chapter 7*	**30 minutes 1 x week** *Wednesday or Friday*						▓		
Sprint 8 *Chapter 8*	**30 minutes 3 x week** *90-95% speed/intensity. 8 reps 70-yards*		▓						
Plyometrics *Chapter 9*	**20 minutes 1 x week** *Tuesday or Saturday*			▓					
Weight Training:	**Exercise:** *Chapter 10*	**Record Sets & Reps Performance** *sets/reps*	*Record amount of weight used during sets in shaded areas.* ***NOTE: Perform E-Lifts*** *(Chp 9) on* ***push & press exercises***						
Chest	Bench press 3/12 Incline press 3/12 Cable flys 3/10 Chest stretch 30 sec	_____ _____ _____	▓						
Back	Pull downs 3/12 T-bar rows 3/12 Up back stretch 30 sec Hyper ext 1/20	_____ _____				▓			
Shoulders	Shoulder press 3/10 Front raises 3/10 Shrugs 3/20 Shoulder stretch 30 sec Rotator cuff 1/15	_____ _____ _____				▓			
Biceps	Curls 3/10 Incl DB curls 3/10	_____						▓	
Triceps	Press downs 3/20 Kick backs 2/20	_____						▓	
Quads	Leg press 3/20 Leg ext 3/20 Lunges 3/10	_____ _____			▓				
Hamstrings	Leg curls 3/20	_____			▓				
Calves	3-way calf raises 3/20 Rev calf raises 1/40	_____			▓				
Abs	Leg raises 3/20 Crunches 2/25	_____				▓		▓	
Obliques	Twists 1/30	_____		▓				▓	

STRATEGIC FITNESS PLAN

Training Log   Level Four   Week 2   Date_____

Workout:	Training Plan:	M	T	W	Th	F	Sat	S
10-Minute Stretching	**4 x week (M, T, Th, Sat)** *Chapter 6*	▨	▨		▨		▨	
Cardio *Chapter 7*	**30 minutes 1 x week** *Wednesday or Friday*					▨		
Sprint 8 *Chapter 8*	**30 minutes 3 x week** *90-95% speed/intensity. 8 reps 70-yards*	▨			▨	▨		
Plyometrics *Chapter 9*	**20 minutes 1 x week** *Tuesday or Saturday*		▨					

Weight Training:	Exercise: *Chapter 10*	Record Sets & Reps Performance *sets/reps*	Record amount of weight used during sets in shaded areas. **NOTE: Perform E-Lifts** (Chp 9) on ***push & press exercises***					

Muscle	Exercise	sets/reps	M	T	W	Th	F	Sat	S
Chest	Bench press Decline press Chest flys Chest stretch	3/12 3/12 3/10 30 sec	▨						
Back	Pull downs Cable rows Up back stretch Hyper ext	3/12 3/12 30 sec 1/20				▨			
Shoulders	Shoulder press Side raises Shrugs Shoulder stretch Rotator cuff	3/10 3/10 3/20 30 sec 2/12				▨			
Biceps	Curls Incl DB curls Forearm curls	3/10 3/10 2/10						▨	
Triceps	Press downs French press	3/20 2/20							
Quads	Leg press Front squats Leg ext	3/20 2/20 3/10		▨					
Hamstrings	Leg curls	3/20		▨					
Calves	3-way calf raises	3/20		▨					
Abs	Leg raises Crunches	3/20 2/25	▨			▨		▨	
Obliques	Side bends	1/30	▨					▨	

STRATEGIC FITNESS PLAN

Training Log   **Level Four**   **Week 3**   **Date_____**

Workout:	Training Plan:		M	T	W	Th	F	Sat	S
10-Minute Stretching	**4 x week (M, T, Th, Sat)** *Chapter 6*		▓	▓		▓		▓	
Cardio *Chapter 7*	**30 minutes 1 x week** *Wednesday or Friday*						▓		
Sprint 8 *Chapter 8*	**30 minutes 3 x week** *90-95% speed/intensity. 8 reps 70-yards*		▓			▓		▓	
Plyometrics *Chapter 9*	**20 minutes 1 x week** *Tuesday or Saturday*			▓					
Weight Training:	**Exercise:** *Chapter 10*	**Record Sets & Reps Performance** *sets/reps*	*Record amount of weight used during sets in shaded areas.* ***NOTE: Perform E-Lifts*** *(Chp 9) on* ***push & press exercises***						
Chest	Bench press 3/12 Incline press 3/12 Chest flys 3/10 Pullovers 1/25 Chest stretch 30 sec	▓	▓						
Back	Pull downs 3/12 T-bar rows 3/12 Up back stretch 30 sec Hyper ext 1/20	▓				▓			
Shoulders	Shoulder press 3/10 Front raises 3/10 Bent laterals 1/15 Shrugs 3/20 Shoulder stretch 30 sec Rotator cuff 2/15	▓				▓			
Biceps	Curls 3/10 Incl DB curls 3/10 Bicep 21s 1 set	▓						▓	
Triceps	Press downs 3/20 Tricep ext 3/20	▓							
Quads	*Leg press* superset 3/10 *Squat jumps* 3/10 Hip Flex 2/10	▓		▓					
Hamstrings	Leg curls 3/20 Stiff dead lift 1/10	▓							
Calves	3-way calf raises 3/20	▓							
Abs	Leg raises 3/20 Crunches 2/25	▓							
Obliques	Twists 1/30	▓							

STRATEGIC FITNESS PLAN

Training Log   **Level Four**   **Week 4**   **Date_____**

Workout:	Training Plan:		M	T	W	Th	F	Sat	S
10-Minute Stretching	**4 x week (M, T, Th, Sat)** *Chapter 6*		▓	▓		▓		▓	
Cardio *Chapter 7*	**30 minutes 1 x week** *Wednesday or Friday*						▓		
Sprint 8 *Chapter 8*	**30 minutes 3 x week** *90-95% speed/intensity. 8 reps 70-yards*		▓						
Plyometrics *Chapter 9*	**20 minutes 1 x week** *Tuesday or Saturday*					▓			

Weight Training:	Exercise: *Chapter 10*	Record Sets & Reps Performance *sets/reps*	*Record amount of weight used during sets in shaded areas.* **NOTE: Perform E-Lifts** *(Chp 9) on* **push & press exercises**						
Chest	Bench press 3/12 Incline press 3/12 Dips 3/10 Pullovers 1/25 Chest stretch 30 sec	_____ _____ _____ _____	▓						
Back	Pull downs 3/12 Cable rows 3/12 Up back stretch 30 sec Hyper ext 1/20	_____ _____							
Shoulders	Sh press 3/10 Side raises 3/10 Bent laterals 3/10 Shrugs 3/20 Shoulder stretch 30 sec Rotator cuff 2/15	_____ _____ _____ _____				▓			
Biceps	Curls 3/10 Incl DB curls 3/10 Bicep 21s 1 set Hammer curls 2/12	_____ _____ _____						▓	
Triceps	Press downs 3/20 Tricep ext 2/15 Rev French press 1/15	_____ _____						▓	
Quads	Leg press 3/20 Hack squats 2/15 One-leg leg ext 3/20 Lunges 2/10	_____ _____ _____							
Hamstrings	Leg curls 3/20								
Calves	3-way calf raises 3/20 Rev calf raises 1/40	_____							
Abs	Leg raises 3/20 Crunches 2/25	_____				▓		▓	
Obliques	Side bends 1/30								

NOTES:

NOTE: Continue the Fitness Plan for this Level until you complete your initial Eight-Week Commitment. For program continuation, additional copies of the Strategic Fitness Plans may be obtained from http://www.readysetgofitness.com/plans.shtml. All purchasers of this book have permission to copy plans for personal use. After the initial eight weeks of training, repeat the Fitness Level adding intensity (more weight, reps, speed), or move to the next Fitness Level.

STRATEGIC FITNESS PLAN
Level Five

MONDAY	TUESDAY	WEDNESDAY	THURSDAY	FRIDAY	SATURDAY	SUNDAY
Warm up Sprints *Chapter 8* **Program A:** 8x60 meters 4x150 meters Alternate with **Program B:** 2-4 sets of: 1x60 meters 1x150 1x300 *(1-2 minutes rest inbetween)* **10-Minute Stretching Routine** *Chapter 6*	Warm up **Plyometrics** 20 minutes *Chapter 9* **Sprints:** 8x40 meters 8x20 **10-Minute Stretching Routine**	*Make-up Day*	Warm up **Plyometrics** 20 minutes **Sprints:** Sprint ladder: 2x60 meters 2x100 2x200 2x100 2x60 **10-Minute Stretching Routine**	**10-Minute Stretching Routine** **Cardio-30** *Chapter 7*	Warm up **Sprints:** 8x10 meters 4X40 4X60 5 sets Bleacher runs and 5 sets of Bleacher Lunges. *walk-down in between* **10-Minute Stretching Routine**	Rest
Weights 1 hour *Chapter 10* 2 hour s 30 minutes	**Weights** 1 hour 2 hours		**Weights** 1 hour 2 hours 30 minutes	**Weights** 1 hour 1 hour 30 minutes	**Weights** 1 hour 2 hours 30 minutes	**TOTAL WEEK TIME:** 11 hours

Level Five is the maximum program designed for off-season, advanced athletes. It's set up for a four-week rotation. Heavy Olympic and power lifting are prescribed for one day a week (*Saturdays*). The weight-training routine is set for five days in the gym. Should you encounter time problems, the following split-routine could be substituted for a four-day-week split: Day 1, chest/back; Day 2, legs; Day 3, shoulders/arms; Day 4, Olympic lifts rotation.

Heavy Olympic and Power Lifting

One day a week, four week rotation

Week 1 Training Plan (Sat)	Performance Weight	sets / reps
Hang Cleans 3 x 3-5		lbs
Squats 5 x 3-5		lbs

Week 2 Training Plan (Sat)	Performance Weight	sets / reps
Push Press 3 x 8-12		lbs
Dead Lifts 5 x 3-5		lbs

Week 3 Training Plan (Sat)	Performance Weight	sets / reps
Hang Cleans 3 x 3-5		lbs
One-Leg Squats 3 x 10		lbs

Week 4 Training Plan (Sat)	Performance Weight	sets / reps
Push Press 3 x 8-12		lbs
Squats 3 x 8		lbs

Level Five is demanding. No, it's very demanding. But it will produce great results! The goal is high-intensity, **injury-free training**. Listen to your body. Injury-free training during the off-season is important in maximizing results. Remember the Isshinryu 90-Percent Extension Rule and E-Lifts (*Chapter 9*).

STRATEGIC FITNESS PLAN

Training Log   **Level Five**   **Week 1**   **Date**_____

Workout:	Training Plan:	M	T	W	Th	F	Sat	S
10-Minute Stretching	**4 x week (M, T, Th, Sat)** *Chapter 6*							
Cardio *Chapter 7*	**30 minutes 2 x week** *Cardio is also multi-tasked with anaerobic training*							
Sprint 8 *Chapter 8*	**30 minutes 3 x week** *90-95% speed/intensity. See Exercise Prescription.*							
Plyometrics *Chapter 9*	**20 minutes 2 x week** *2 sets plyo-drills*							

Weight Training:	**Exercise:** *Chapter 10*	**Record Sets & Reps Performance** *sets/reps*	*Record amount of weight used during sets in shaded areas.* **NOTE: Perform E-Lifts** *(Chp 9)* on **push & press exercises**					
Chest	Bench press 3/8 Incline press 3/12 Cable chest press 3/10 Cable flys 3/10 Chest stretch 30 sec	_____ _____ _____ _____ _____						
Back	Pull downs 5/12 Dumbbell rows 3/12 Up back stretch 30 sec Hyper ext 2/15	_____ _____ _____ _____						
Shoulders	Sh press 5/8 Front raises 3/10 Bent laterals 3/10 Shrugs 3/20 Shoulder stretch 30 sec Rotator cuff 2/15	_____ _____ _____ _____ _____						
Biceps	Curls 5/10 Incl DB curls 3/10 Bicep 21s 3 sets Forearm curls 2/10	_____ _____ _____ _____						
Triceps	Press downs 3/20 Kick backs 3/20 Rev press downs 3/15	_____ _____ _____						
Quads	*Leg press* superset 3/10 *Squat jumps* 3/10 Lunges 3/10 Leg ext 3/20	_____ _____ _____ _____						
Hamstrings	Leg curls 3/10 Stiff leg dead lift 1/10	_____ _____						
Calves	3-way calf raises 3/20 Rev calf raises 1/50	_____ _____						
Abs	Leg raises 3/20 Crunches 2/20	_____						
Obliques	Side bends 1/30							

Heavy power lifting on Saturday

STRATEGIC FITNESS PLAN

Training Log   Level Five   Week 2   Date_____

Workout:	Training Plan:	M	Tu	W	Th	F	Sat	S
10-Minute Stretching	**4 x week (M, T, Th, Sat)** *Chapter 6*							
Cardio *Chapter 7*	**30 minutes 2 x week**							
Sprint 8 *Chapter 8*	**30 minutes 3 x week** *90-95% speed/intensity*							
Plyometrics *Chapter 9*	**20 minutes 2 x week** *2 sets plyo-drills*							

Weight Training:	**Exercise:** *Chapter 10*	**Record Sets & Reps Performance** *sets/reps*	*Record amount of weight used during sets in shaded areas.* ***NOTE: Perform E-Lifts** (Chp 9) on **push & press exercises***					
Chest	Bench press 3/8 Incline press 3/12 Decline press 3/10 D/B flys 3/10 Pullovers 1/25 Chest stretch 30 sec	_____ _____ _____ _____ _____						*Heavy power lifting on Saturday*
Back	Pull downs 5/12 Cable rows 3/12 Up back stretch 30 sec Hyper ext 2/20	_____ _____						
Shoulders	Sh press 5/5 Side raises 3/10 Bent laterals 3/10 Shrugs 3/20 Shoulder stretch 30 sec Rotator cuff 2/15	_____ _____ _____ _____						
Biceps	Curls 5/10 Incl DB curls 3/10 Bicep 21s 3 sets Hammer curls 2/10	_____ _____ _____						
Triceps	Press downs 3/20 Tricep ext 3/20 Kick backs 3/15	_____ _____						
Quads	*Leg press* superset 3/10 *Squat jumps* 3/10 Hack squats 3/10 Hip flexors Rev 2/10	_____ _____ _____						
Hamstrings	Leg curls 5/8	_____						
Calves	3-way calf raises 6/20							
Abs	Leg raises 3/25 Crunches 2/30	_____						
Obliques	Twists 1/30							

STRATEGIC FITNESS PLAN

Training Log   **Level Five**   **Week 3**   **Date_____**

Workout:	Training Plan:		M	T	W	Th	F	Sat	S
10-Minute Stretching	**4 x week (M, T, Th, Sat)** *Chapter 6*		▨	▨		▨		▨	
Cardio *Chapter 7*	**30 minutes 2 x week**				▨		▨		
Sprint 8 *Chapter 8*	**30 minutes 3 x week** *90-95% speed/intensity*			▨		▨		▨	
Plyometrics *Chapter 9*	**20 minutes 2 x week** *2 sets plyo-drills*			▨		▨			
Weight Training:	**Exercise:** *Chapter 10*	**Record Sets & Reps Performance** *sets/reps*	*Record amount of weight used during sets in shaded areas.* **NOTE: Perform E-Lifts** *(Chp 9)* on **push & press exercises**						

Chest	Bench press 3/8 / Incline press 3/12 / Cable chest press 3/10 / Cable flys 3/10 / Chest stretch 30 sec	▨ (Heavy power lifting on Saturday)

Heavy power lifting on Saturday

Chest	Bench press	3/8
	Incline press	3/12
	Cable chest press	3/10
	Cable flys	3/10
	Chest stretch	30 sec
Back	Pull downs	5/12
	Cable rows	3/12
	Up back stretch	30 sec
	Hyper ext	2/20
Shoulders	Sh press	5/8
	Front raises	3/10
	Bent laterals	3/10
	Shrugs	3/20
	Shoulder stretch	30 sec
	Rotator cuff	2/15
Biceps	Curls	5/10
	Incl DB curls	3/10
	Bicep 21s	3 sets
	Forearm curls	2/10
Triceps	Press downs	3/20
	French press	3/20
	Rev press downs	1/15
Quads	Leg press	3/20
	One-leg squats	3/10
	Leg ext	3/20
	Hip flexors	3/10
Hamstrings	Leg curls	3/10
	Stiff leg dead lift	1/10
Calves	3-way calf raises	3/20
	Rev calf raises	1/50
Abs	Leg raises	3/25
	Crunches	2/30
Obliques	Side bends	1/30

STRATEGIC FITNESS PLAN

Training Log   Level Five   Week 4   Date_____

Workout:	Training Plan:		M	Tu	W	Th	F	Sat	S
10-Minute Stretching	**4 x week (M, T, Th, Sat)** *Chapter 6*		▓	▓		▓		▓	
Cardio *Chapter 7*	**30 minutes 2 x week**				▓		▓		
Sprint 8 *Chapter 8*	**30 minutes 3 x week** *90-95% speed/intensity*		▓			▓		▓	
Plyometrics *Chapter 9*	**20 minutes 2 x week** *2 sets plyo-drills*		▓			▓			
Weight Training:	**Exercise:** *Chapter 10*	**Record Sets & Reps Performance** *sets/reps*		*Record amount of weight used during sets in shaded areas.* **NOTE: Perform E-Lifts** *(Chp 9)* on **push & press exercises**					

Weight Training:	Exercise:		Record Sets & Reps Performance	M	Tu	W	Th	F	Sat	S
Chest	Bench press Incline press Dips Cable flys Pullovers Chest stretch	3/8 3/12 3/10 3/10 1/25 30 sec	_____ _____ _____ _____ _____ _____	▓					*Heavy power lifting on Saturday*	
Back	Pull downs T-bar rows Up back stretch Hyper ext	5/12 3/12 30 sec 2/20	_____ _____ _____ _____				▓			
Shoulders	Sh press Side raises Bent laterals Shrugs Shoulder stretch Rotator cuff	5/5 3/10 3/10 3/20 30 sec 2/15	_____ _____ _____ _____ _____ _____		▓		▓			
Biceps	Curls Incl DB curls Bicep 21s Hammer curls	5/10 3/10 3 sets 2/10	_____ _____ _____ _____					▓		
Triceps	Press downs French press Rev press downs	3/20 3/20 3/15	_____ _____ _____							
Quads	*Leg press* superset *Squat jumps* front squats One-leg leg ext	3/10 3/10 3/10 3/10	_____ _____ _____ _____		▓					
Hamstrings	Leg curls	5/8	_____							
Calves	3-way calf raises	6/20	_____							
Abs	Leg raises Crunches	3/25 2/30	_____				▓		▓	
Obliques	Twists	1/30	_____		▓					

NOTES:

Conclusion

The single most important aspect of health and fitness improvement is discussed in this conclusion.

This one aspect cannot be sold in a nutrition store, obtained with a physician's prescription pad, or purchased at a gym. The single most important aspect of fitness improvement is absolutely free.

This issue is so fundamental that even with the medical research information from this book and a Strategic Fitness Plan as a guide, this one aspect will ultimately determine the success of your fitness program.

If not accomplished, this one issue stands in the way of achieving a new appearance, feeling great about yourself, and raising your health and fitness to new levels. The most important fitness component is the *commitment you make* to follow a Strategic Fitness Plan for the first eight weeks.

During the first eight weeks, you'll need 100 percent determination to stay with your Strategic Fitness Plan.

While this book was written to be a lifelong exercise prescription, short-range goals help determine if we are on the correct course towards our long-range objectives.

The first eight-week period is critically important and will determine the success of your fitness improvement effort.

Researchers demonstrate that signing a statement of commitment expressing intent to train will significantly increase success.

(Facilitating changes in exercise behavior: effect of structured statements of intention on perceived barriers to action, 1995, Huddy).

Researchers show there are several key factors that might keep you from making a serious commitment to begin, and stick with, a total fitness program: perceived barriers, past experience, or fear of failure or embarrassment (*Use of attitude-behavior models in exercise promotion*, 1990, Godin).

These are natural human emotions that need to be worked through. And the best way to do this is simply by understanding that these are natural feelings felt by everyone beginning a new program.

A research test group that had signed a structured *"statement of intent for an exercise plan"* that addressed "major barriers" had a two-fold increase in frequency and intensity of exercise over the group that did not sign the statement.

At the end of the following discussion concerning what happens during the first eight weeks of training, there is a commitment form you should seriously consider signing. This will formalize your eight-week commitment - to you! No one else. This commitment form is for you . . only!

Major Barriers

Major barriers that might deter you from achieving your commitment should be thought through, and action plans to overcome each barrier should be developed before signing.

These barriers might be work schedule, family responsibility, travel schedule, and gym or home equipment availability. Develop a specific action plan to deal with each barrier.

SYNERGY FITNESS STRATEGY 10

Make the Eight-Week Commitment

The First Eight Weeks

Psychologists tell us, that when starting something new (like a new fitness program), initially we are enthusiastic. Then we go through four phases before the new activity becomes internalized and becomes part of who we are as individuals. The four phases are **Form**, **Storm**, **Norm**, and **Perform**.

The *Form* phase is marked with the excitement of beginning a new program. During the first week of your fitness plan, sticking with the plan should be easy. You may even feel you can handle more training. Don't do this. Not only does overtraining risk injury, it risks your motivation and continuation of the fitness program over time.

One main mental deterrent occurs during this phase - waiting for all the lights to turn green before beginning. While preparation is good, pick a start date, go for it, and don't look back.

The *Storm* phase follows a few weeks later. When we learn the program is hard work (on some days), and we just don't want to train - this is the storm phase. It happens to everyone.

In the *Storm* phase, we begin to create excuses (conscious and subconscious) for missing workouts. This is, by far, the toughest phase.

How should you get through this phase? Mentally prepare ahead of time. The *Storm* phase is a natural phase that everyone experiences. And the key to overcoming it is to make the commitment now to press through the bad weather of the *Storm* phase. And this will happen. Plan on it! Just don't let this natural human emotion deter you from reaching your fitness goals.

Researchers show that dieters who were dissatisfied with their bodies only have a 36 percent success rate with a diet and exercise program. Dieters more satisfied with their bodies have a 63 percent success rate. (Characteristics of successful and unsuccessful dieters: an application of signal detection methodology, 1998, Kiernan).

Consistency is a must during the initial eight weeks. Following your Fitness Plan will improve appearance and produce fitness gains rapidly. The positive results will increase satisfaction and motivation to continue.

The *Norm* phase is adapting to your fitness training commitment by learning that you can press through the tough days when you do not feel like training and still get in a great workout. Every successful, long-term training individual knows - feeling bad at the beginning of the workout often means this will be the best workout of the week.

The *Perform* phase occurs when you have experienced the first three phases and begin to train consistently. It's when fitness training becomes internalized.

Repetition eventually becomes habit. Training can't be a choice. Fitness training is just something that you do because you are you! Training must become a part of who you are. This is the *Perform* phase.

During the first eight weeks, you will not only be making positive physical changes, but you will also be having positive mental changes as well.

Don't make the mistake of thinking that you will bypass the first three phases and go straight to the *Perform* phase. This is a mistake. When this happens, the *Storm* phase seems forcefully to pop up and pull the person back into this phase for a few body slams before letting go.

A better strategy is simply to be mentally prepared for all four phases *in advance.* Identify the phase you are experiencing, and, with maturity and confidence, work through the mental aspects of training by sticking to the plan on the tough days.

When you reach the *Perform* phase, maintaining the fitness plan is much easier. But you can't get there until the first eight weeks are completed. Completing the Fitness Success Plan work sheet (*right*) will be helpful.

Fitness Success Plan

Barriers to the success of following your Strategic Fitness Plan for eight weeks:

Action plans to overcome barriers:

It is time to make the Eight Week Commitment. This is a private, but formal promise . . . to you . . . that you will follow your Strategic Fitness Plan consistently for eight weeks.

We're not thinking about long-term yet. Just focus on the first eight weeks for now.

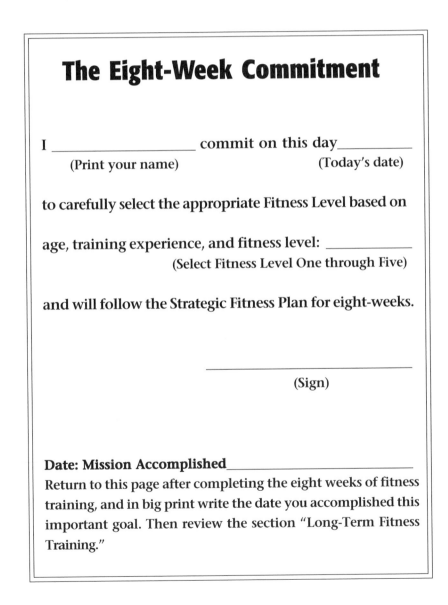

The Eight-Week Commitment

I _____ commit on this day_____
   (Print your name)   (Today's date)

to carefully select the appropriate Fitness Level based on

age, training experience, and fitness level: _____
                                 (Select Fitness Level One through Five)

and will follow the Strategic Fitness Plan for eight-weeks.

_____
                   (Sign)

Date: Mission Accomplished_____
Return to this page after completing the eight weeks of fitness training, and in big print write the date you accomplished this important goal. Then review the section "Long-Term Fitness Training."

Long-Term Fitness Training

The key to long-term training is to be aware that motivation comes and goes, and comes and goes.

The one day that you decide to miss could be the last workout for a year. Long-term training is not a physical issue; it is a mental one.

I have a mental practice that I use to help me through the tough days when I do not feel like training. I don't make the decision to miss a workout until I first change into my training clothes.

If I decide to miss a workout, that is okay (sometimes it's unavoidable), but I always make the effort to change clothes first.

Most of the time, just changing into training clothes is enough to get me started. Once started, this typically becomes the best workout of the week.

Researchers show that lifelong exercise can counteract the effects associated with aging of the neuromuscular system. (Effects of strength and endurance training on skeletal muscles in the elderly. New muscles for old! 1999, Lexell).

Why People Stop Exercising

Everyone who has stopped exercising began by "missing once." That one miss led to another, then another. The key to long-term training is to understand the mental risk associated with missing "one workout."

I can't overemphasize the importance of mentally making an issue of missing "one workout."

Missing one workout will not hurt you physically. Mentally, however, missing a workout permanently breaks the habit of training - until you make the next workout.

When deciding to miss, tell yourself that you just decided to "stop training permanently" - until you have completed the next workout.

Ten Ready, Set, Go! Fitness Strategies

The health and fitness information presented in this book is reliable. It's supported by biomedical research and will produce positive results.

Whether you are a physician writing an "exercise prescription" for patients, a triathlete looking to reduce time per mile and build strength in key areas for injury prevention, an athlete training for the upcoming season, a bodybuilder seeking to improve symmetry by reducing percentage of body fat while adding lean muscle, or middle-aged and wanting to get into shape - following one of the five Strategic Fitness Plans in the preceding chapter will help you achieve your fitness goals.

In reading this book, you have seen Ten Fitness Strategies. They are worth reviewing periodically.

Ready, Set, Go! Fitness Strategies

1. **Increase growth hormone naturally**

2. **Reach HGH release benchmarks during fitness training**
   · Out-of-breath (oxygen debt)
   · Muscle burn (lactic acid)
   · Increased body temperature
   · Adrenal response (slightly painful)

3. **Maximize HGH release during fitness training**

   Before training: No high fat meals one hour prior

                            Intake some carbs to fuel intensity

   During training: Drink lots of water

   After training: Limit sugar for two hours

                            Intake 25 grams of protein

4. **Get adequate deep sleep**

5. **Take 2-grams of L-glutamine before fitness training**

6. **Maintain insulin balance with a balanced diet / in moderation**

7. **Use The Target Zone Training Method by targeting slow, fast, and super-fast muscle fiber during training**

8. **Use a comprehensive strategic fitness plan to increase flexibility, endurance, anaerobic capacity, strength, and power**

9. **During resistance training, isolate muscles being worked, train every set to exhaustion, aerobically with E-Lifts on push and press exercises**

10. **Make the Eight-Week Commitment**

Concluding Thoughts

Many Olympic athletes are thought to be near, or at the end of their competitive days, by age 30. This view of competition is limited and narrow. And it's harmful.

The current definition of competition leads athletes to secretly hide the use of steroids and other illegal substances that enhance performance because society thinks competition is about winning at all costs.

Don't misunderstand. I love competition. And I believe the national health problem is due to the lack of meaningful competition for all ages.

Competition should be, and could be, a tool for health improvement.

We have the Senior Olympics and the Special Olympics. What we need is the Masters Olympics for ages 30 and up (with incentives for as many participants as possible).

Most people stop competing in physical events after high school. A small number continue in college through intramurals. Unless you are in that very small number making it to the professional ranks, almost all competition is over - for life - after high school.

This view of competition leaves us with essentially "slow-twitch" muscle developing competitions - with perhaps tennis and softball being the exceptions. The only widespread competitions available are marathons. However, the amount of training time required makes this event impractical for most people with active careers and children to raise.

Most are unaware of master's competitions in swimming, cycling, XC skiing, and track and field.

Competition can be a tool for good health, or it can be harmful. On the news, we see parents fill their missing need for competition by fighting and injuring others during their children's games.

As a nation, we need to create healthy and meaningful competition for adults of all ages.

The physical benefits of maintaining competition throughout life would be enormous. In my humble opinion, this would help to cure the nation's health problem.

Actively practicing physicians must move to a leadership role in curing the national health problem by setting the example and encouraging others to begin fitness training.

Educators, seeing obesity at epidemic rates, need to take a leadership role and find the balance between test scores and fitness scores of their students. Public health officials, often overwhelmed with endless paperwork requirements, need to take a proactive role.

We have health information everywhere, but it's not working. In fact, we could produce a chart showing health information climbing and health status going down. Producing more reports is not the answer.

Motivation is what we need. And a new model that views competition as a tool could start a fitness improvement revival.

Sports for Life

Competition for middle-aged and older adults could provide additional motivation for many. Rather than telling people to lose weight and exercise, perhaps encouragement to begin training for a 200-meter race for the next Senior Olympics competition or masters event would provide additional motivation.

It was once thought that a selective loss of fast-twitch muscle fiber occurred naturally with aging. New research shows that this is not true. Fitness training - even at ages above 70 years - can develop fast-twitch muscle fiber that is necessary for anaerobic, growth hormone producing exercise.

Researchers demonstrate that older men (age 52-62) experience a decrease of type II muscle fiber during aging; however, training can prevent this effect of aging, (Oxidative capacity of human muscle fiber types: effects of age and training status, 1995, Proctor).

Decreased physical activity with aging appears to be the key factor involved in muscle wasting (Sarcopenia, 2001, Morley).

Researchers show that muscle wasting (sarcopenia) is implicated with the decrease of HGH during aging. This condition occurs with a "disproportionate wasting (atrophy) of fast-twitch muscle fibers." In short, if we do not continue to use all three muscle fiber types during exercise, we will lose the capacity to increase the body's ability to produce exercise-induced growth hormone - because we no longer have fast-twitch muscle fiber that is necessary for anaerobic exercise.

Researchers prove that older men (average age 74) could increase muscle cell size, strength, velocity of movement, and power in both slow and fast-twitch muscle fiber (*Effect of resistance training on single muscle fiber contractile function in older men,* 2000, Trappe).

This research also demonstrates that fast-twitch fiber is not activated until the exercise reaches a certain level of high-intensity effort - that we are missing without competition.

Clearly, there's a huge need for leadership that will develop widespread competitions for adults with emphasis on fast-twitch muscle development like masters track and field, swimming, XC skiing, and cycling. And there should be more support for Senior Games and the Senior Olympics.

Inactivity is a natural part of aging?

Wrong!

This attitude may be responsible for thousands of premature deaths and the U.S. health crisis

The Take Home

As we age, the absence of healthy competition and the lack of comprehensive fitness training - that includes anaerobic exercise - causes significant health and fitness problems.

If you were to look through a microscope at your muscle cells during youth, you would see a uniformity of cells and the proper distribution of muscle fibers - slow, fast, and super-fast.

Looking at older muscles under a microscope, you would see some uniformity with the slow muscle fiber along with an unorganized group of fast-twitch muscle cells. Due to inactivity, these cells decreased in size and strength.

To maintain fitness for a lifetime, it is not sufficient to exercise in the traditional manner. Jogging will develop your slow-twitch muscle fiber in your legs. Bench press performed in the traditional slow tempo will strengthen the slow muscle fiber in your chest.

To achieve optimum fitness (and maintain it during aging), you will need to begin a new way of thinking, a new paradigm, if you will, about health, fitness, and aging.

The thinking needs to be focused on the question - *how do I develop and maintain the three types of muscle fiber - so I can have a body that can handle high-intensity, anaerobic, growth hormone releasing exercise - for a lifetime?*

The Strategic Fitness Plan for your appropriate Fitness Level will accomplish *The Target Zone Training* and develop the different muscle fiber in your body. And the anaerobic workouts will release the most powerful fitness improving hormone into your body.

The New Fitness Paradigm

Are we entering a new paradigm of health and fitness? It's too early to tell. But there's hope.

Hot-off-the-press biomedical research certainly supports the need for a comprehensive fitness training model that includes (the missing ingredient) anaerobic exercise.

The better question may be - how long will it take before physicians begin writing "exercise prescriptions" for their patients for comprehensive fitness training? Or, how long will it be before a major national focus is placed on creating widespread athletic competition for middle-aged adults?

There have been two major worldwide fitness revolutions - weightlifting in the 1960s and distance running in the 1980s.

Famous U.S. weightlifting coach Bob Hoffman began promoting resistance training and endorsing weight lifting equipment in the 1960s. This movement caught fire, and today in the United States, there are 16,000 fitness centers and health clubs, which is up by 4,000 in recent years. Fitness centers are located in nearly every city across the country.

Home cardio equipment and home strength training units are being purchased at record numbers.

Many participated in the "cardio" revolution in the 1980s. Dr. Kenneth Cooper wrote the book *Aerobics* and fired the starting gun for the world to begin jogging. And we began believing quality of life could be enhanced by performing aerobic exercise.

Many benefited from the aerobics and weight training national movements. However, it is time to implement a new comprehensive fitness training model that includes high-intensity anaerobic training for children and adults of all ages.

We have a national health fitness crisis. And you have the cure. Don't keep it to yourself.

I hope you will become a leader and solve this problem by encouraging family members, friends, and neighbors to join you in your commitment to improve fitness. Most of all, it is my hope that you will implement the information presented in this book and improve your health, fitness, and appearance beyond your wildest imagination.

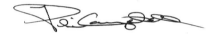

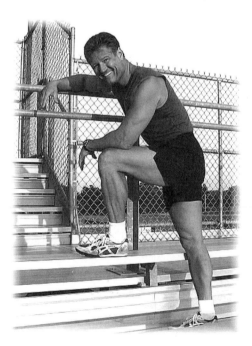

References

Many references have citations placed in the text or a Research Box near the topic.

Introduction & Chapter 1

Atalay, Sen. (1999). "Physical exercise and antioxidant defenses in the heart."
    Ann N Y Sci. Jun30;874:169-77. PMID: 10415530.

Biolo, Maggi, Williams, Tipton, Wolfe. (1995). "Increased rates of muscle protein turnover
    and amino acid transport after resistance exercise in humans." *Am J Physiol.*
    Mar;268(3 Pt 1):E514-20. PMID: 7900797.

Cappon, Ipp, Brasel, Cooper. (1993). "Acute effects of high fats and high glucose meals on
    the growth hormone response to exercise." *J Clin Endocrinol Metab.* Jun;76(6):1418-
    22. PMID: 8501145.

Cheung, Zhao, Chait, Albers, Brown. (2001). "Antioxidant supplements block the response
    of hdl to simvastatin-niacin therapy in patients with coronary artery disease and low
    hdl." *Arterioscler Thromb Vasc Biol.* Aug;21(8):1320-6. PMID: 11498460.

Christensen, Jorgensen, Moller, Orskov. (1984). "Characterization of growth hormone
    release in response to external heating. Comparison to exercise induced release."
    Acta Endocrinol. Nov;107(3):295-301. PMID: 6507003.

Chwalbinski-Moneta. (1996). "Threshold increases in plasma growth hormone in
    relation to plasma catecholamine and blood lactate concentration during
    progressive exercise in endurance-trained athletes."
    Eur J Appl Physiol Occup Physiol. 73(1-2):117-20. PMID: 8861679.

Di Luigi, Guidetti, Nordio, Baldari, Romanelli. (2001). "Acute effect of physical
    exercise on serum insulin-like growth factor-binding protein 2 and 3 in
    healthy men: role of exercise linked growth hormone secretion."
    Int J Sports Med. Feb;22(2):103-110. PMID: 11291611.

Di Luigi, Guidetti, Pigozzi, Baldari, Casini, Nordio, Romanelli. (1999). "Acute
    amino Acids supplementation enhances pituitary responsiveness in athletics."
    Med Sci Sports Exerc. Dec;31(12):1748-54. PMID: 10613424.

Eberhardt, Ingram, Makuc. (2001). Urban and Rural Health Chartbook. *Health,
    United States, 2001.* Hyattsville, Maryland: National Center for Health Statistics.

Elias, Wilson, Naqvi, Pandan. (1997). "Effects of blood pH and blood lactate on
    growth hormone, prolactin, and gonadotropin release after acute exercise in
    male volunteers. *Proc Soc Exp Biol Med.* Feb;214(2):156-60. PMID: 9034133.

Felsing, Brasel, Cooper. (1992). "Effect of low and high intensity exercise on
    circulating growth hormone in men. *J Clin Endocrinol Metab.*
    Jul;75(1):157-62. PMID: 1619005.

Frewin, Frantz, Downey. (1976). "The effect of ambient temperature on the growth hormone and prolactin response to exercise." *Aust J Exp Biol Med Sci.* Feb:54(1):97-101. PMID: 942365.

Groussard, Morel, Chevanne, Monnier, Cillard, Delamarche. (2000). Free radical scavenging and antioxidant effects of lactate ion: an in vitro study." *J Appl Physiol.* Jul;89(1):169-75. PMID: 10904049.

Kastello, Sothmann, Murthy. (1993). "Young and old subjects for aerobic capacity have similar noradrenergic responses to exercise." *J Appl Physiol.* Jan;74(1):49-54. PMID: 8444733.

Lemura, Von Duvillard, Mookerjee. (2000). "The effects of physical training on functional capacity in adults. Ages 46 to 90: a meta-analysis." *J Sports Med Phy Fitness.* Mar;40(1):1-10. PMID: 10822903.

Lugar. (1988). "Acute exercise stimulates the rennin-angiotensin-aldosterone axis adaptive changes in runners." *Horm Res.* 30(1);5-9. PMID: 2851526.

Meirleir, Naaktgeboren. (1986). "Beta-endorphin and ACTH levels in peripheral blood during and after aerobic and anaerobic exercise." *Eur J Appl Physiol Occup Physiol.* 55(1):5-8. PMID: 3009176.

MacIntyre, Reid, McKenzie. (1995). "Delayed muscle soreness. The inflammatory response to muscle injury and its clinical implications." *Sports Med.* Jul;20(1):24-40. PMID: 7481277.

Paw, De Jong, Pallast, Kloek, Schouten, Kok. (2000). "Immunity in frail elderly: a randomized controlled trial of exercise and enriched foods." *Med Sci Sports Exerc.* Dec:32(12):2005-11. PMID: 11128843.

Parise, Yarasheski. (2000). "The utility of resistance training and amino acid supplementation for reversing age-associated decrements in muscle protein mass and function." *Curr Opin Clin Nutr Metab Care.* Nov 3;(6):489-95. PMID:11085836.

Peyreigne, Bouix, Fedou, Mercier. (2001). "Effect of hydration on exercise-induced growth hormone." *Eur J Endocrinol.* Sept;145(4):445-50. PMID: 115810003.

Pritzlaff, Wideman, Weltman, J., Abbott, Gutgesell, Hartman, Veldhuis, Weltman, A. (2000). "Catecholamine release, growth hormone secretion, and energy expenditure during exercise vs. recovery in men." *J Appl Physiol.* Sept;89(3):937-46. PMID: 10956336.

Pritzlaff, Wideman, Weltman, J., Abbott, Gutgesell, Hartman, Veldhuis, Weltman, A. (2000). "Impact of acute exercise intensity on pulsatile growth hormone release in men." *J Appl Physiol.* Aug;87(2):498-504. PMID: 10444604.

Sutton, Lazarus. (1976). "Growth hormone in exercise: comparison of physiological and pharmacological stimuli." *J Appl Physiol.* Oct;41(4):523-7. PMID: 985395.

Stokes, Nevill, Hall Lakomy. (2002). "Growth Hormone responses to repeated maximal cycle ergometer exercise at different pedaling rates." J Appl Physiol 2992 Feb;92(2):602-8 PMID: 11796670

Terry, Willoughby, Braseau, Martin, Patel. (1976). "Antiserum to somatostatin prevents stress-induced inhibition of growth hormone secretion in the rat." *Science.* May 7;192(4239):565-7. PMID: 1257793.

Toogood, O'Neill, Shalet. (1996). "Beyond the somatopause: growth hormone deficiency in adults over the age of 60 years." *J Clin Endocrinol Metab.* Feb; 81(2):460-5. National Library of Science, PubMed abstract: 8636250.

Vanhelder, Radomski, Goode. (1984). "Growth hormone responses during intermittent weightlifting exercise in Men." *Eur J Physiol Occup Physiol.* 53(1):31-4. PMID: 6542499.

Vigas, Celko, Koska. (2000). "Role of body temperature in exercise-induced growth hormone and prolactin release in non-trained and physically fit subjects." Endocr Regul. Dec;34(4):175-180. PMID: 11137977.

Weltman, Weltman, Womack, Davis, Blumer, Gasser, Hartman. (1997). "Exercise training decreases the growth hormone (GH) response to acute constant-load exercise." *Med Sci Sports Exer. May;29(5):660-76.*

Weltman, Pritzlaff, Wideman, Blumer, Abbott, Hartman, Veldhuis. (2000). "Exercise-dependent growth hormone release is linked to markers of heightened central adrenergic outflow." *J Appl Physiol.* Aug;89(2):629-35.

Wideman, Weltman, Patrie. (2000). "Synergy of L-arginine and GHRP-2 stimulation of growth hormone in men and women: modulation by exercise." *Applied Journal of Physiology.* Oct;279(4) R1467-77.

Wideman L, Weltman, Shah, Story, Veldhuis, Weltman A. (1999). "Effects of gender on exercise-induced growth hormone release." *J Appl Physiol.* Sept;87(3):1154-62. PMID: 10484590.

Zhang, Guoyu, Irwin. (2000). "Utilization of preventative medical services in the United States: a comparison between rural and urban populations." *J Rural Health.* Fall;16(4):349-56.

Chapters 2 & 3

Booth, Gordon, Carlson, Hamilton. (2000). "Waging war on modern chronic diseases: primary prevention through exercise biology." *J Appl Physiol.* Feb;88(2):774-87. PMID: 10658050.

Calabresi, Ishikawa, Bartolini. (1996). "Somatostatin infusion suppresses GH secretory burst frequency and mass in normal men." *American Journal of Physiology.* Jun;270(6 Pt1):E975-9. PMID: 8764181.

Chein, Vogt, Terry. (1999). "Clinical experiences using a low-dose, high frequency human growth hormone treatment regimen." *Journal of Advancement in Medicine.* 12(3). www.drchein.com.

Colao, Marzullo, Spiezia. (1999). "Effect of growth hormone and insulin like growth factor on prostate diseases: An ultrasonographic and endocrine study in Acromegaly, GH deficiency, and healthy subjects." *J. Clinical Endocrinol Metab.* 84:1986-91.

Corpas, Harman, Blackman. (1993). Human growth hormone and human aging." *Endocrinol Review,* Feb; 14(1):20-39. National Library of Medicine, PubMed: 8491152.

D'Costa, Ingram, Lenham, Sonntag. (1993). "The regulation and mechanism of Action of growth hormone and insulin-like growth factor 1 during normal aging." *Journal of Reproductive Fertil Suppl:*46:87-98. National Library of Science, PubMed abstract: 8636250.

Jenkins. (1999). "Growth hormone and exercise." *Clin Endocrinol (Oxf).* Jun;50(6):683-9. PMID: 10468938.

Kiernan, King, Kraemer, Stefanick, Killen. (2000). "Characteristics of successful dieters: an application of signal detection methodology." *Ann Behav Med.* Winter;20(1):1-6.PMID: 9755345.

Kraemer, Newton. (2000). "Training for muscular power." *Phys Med Rehabil Clin Am.* May11;(2):341-68. PMID: 10810765.

Gibney, Wallace, Spinks. (1999). "The effects of 10 years of recombinant growth hormone (GH) in adult GH-deficient patients." *J Clin Endocrinol Metab.* 84:2596-2602.

Goji, K. (1993). "Pulsatile characteristics of spontaneous growth hormone (GH) concentration profiles in boys evaluated by an ultrasensitive immunoradiometric assay: evidence for ultradian periodicity of GH secretion." *J Clinical Endocrinology Metabolism.* Mar;76(3):667-70.

Jamieson, Dorman, with Valerie Marriott. *(1997). Growth Hormone: Reversing the Aging Process Naturally. The Methuselah Factor.* East Canaan, Connecticut: SAFE GOODS in conjunction with Longevity News Network.

Lieberman, Hoffman. (1997). "The somatopause: should growth hormone deficiency in older people be treated?" *Clinical Geriatric Medicine.* Nov:13(4):671-84. PMID: 9354748.

Nicklas, Ryan, Treuth, Harman, Blackman, Hurley, Rogers. (1995). "Testosterone, growth hormone and IGF-1 responses to Acute and chronic resistive exercise in man aged 55-70 years." *Int Journal Sports Medicine*, Oct;16(7):445-50. National Library of Science, PubMed abstract: 8550252.

Oldenburg, Ann. (2000). "The fountain of youth flows from a needle." *USA Today.* Nov. 14, 2000.

Pfeifer, Verhovec, Zizek. (1999). "Growth hormone treatment reverses early atherosclerotic changes in GH deficient adults." *J Clin Endocrinol Metab.* 84:453-457.

Rudman, Daniel, and colleagues. (1990). "Effects of human growth hormone in men over 60 years old." *New England Journal of Medicine,* Volume, 323, July 5, 1990, Number 1.

Snibson, Bhathal, Adams. (2001). "Overexpressed growth hormone (GH) synergistically promotes carcinogen-initiated liver tumour growth by promoting cellular proliferation in emerging hepatocellular neoplasms in female and male GH-transgenic mice. *Liver.* Apr;21(2):149-58. PMID: 11318985.

Sports Club Association Newsletter, *International Health Racket.* Nov. 2000.

Takala, Ruokonen, Webster. (1999). "Increased mortality associated with growth hormone treatment in critically III adults." *N Eng J Med* 341:785-92.

Toogood, Shalet. (1998). "Aging and growth hormone." *Baillieres Clinical Endocrinology Metabolism*, July: 12 (2):281-96. National Library of Science, PubMed abstract: 10083897.

Toogood, O'Neill, Shalet. (1996). "Beyond the somatopause: growth hormone deficiency in adults over the age of 60 years." *J Clin Endocrinol Metabol.* Feb; 81(2):460-5. National Library of Science, PubMed abstract: 8636250.

Van Buul-Offers, Kooijman. (1998) "The role of growth hormone and insulin-like growth factors in the immune system." *Cell Mol Life Science,* Oct; 54(10): 1083-94. National Library of Science, PubMed abstract: 9817987.

Winer, Shaw, Baumann. (1990). "Basal plasma growth hormone levels in man: new evidence for rhythmicity of growth hormone secretion." *J Clinical Endocrinology Metabolism.* Jun;70(6):1678-86. PMID: 2347901.

Ames, BN. (2001). "DNA damage from micronutrient deficiencies is likely to be a major cause of cancer." *Mutat Res.* Apr 18;475(1-2):7-20. PMID: 11205149.

Bewaerets, Moorkens, Abs. (1998). "Secretion of growth hormone in patients with chronic fatigue syndrome." *Growth Hormone IGF Res*, April 8, Suppl B: 127-9. Washington, D.C., National Library of Medicine, PMID: 10990147.

Bruls, Crasson, Van Reeth, Legros. (2000). "Melatonin. II. Physiological and therapeutic effects." *Rev Med Liege.* Sept;55(9):862-70. PMID: 11105602.

Carranza-Lira, Garcia. (2000). "Melatonin and climactery." *Med Sci Monit.* Nov-Dec;6(6):1209-12. PMID: 11208481.

Casabiell, Gualillo, Pombo, Dieguez, Casanueva. (1999). "Growth hormone secretagogues: the clinical future." *Horm Res* 1999;51 Suppl 3:29-33. National Library of Science, PubMed abstract: 10592441.

Colgan, Michael. (1993). *Optimum Sports Nutrition, Your Competitive Edge.* New York, NY. Advanced Research Press.

Centers for Disease Control and Prevention. (2000). "Diabetes, A Serious Public Health Problem, AT-A-GLANCE 2000." *Diabetes Public Health Resource.* Atlanta, Georgia. March 9, 2000.

Centers for Disease Control and Prevention. (2000). "CDC: Diabetes, obesity becoming epidemic." *AP News.* January 25,2001. www.Healthcentral.com.

Cox, Cortright, Dohm, Houmard. (1999). "Effect of aging on response to Exercise training in humans: skeletal muscle GLUT-4 and insulin sensitivity." *J Applied Physiology.* June;86(6):2019-25.

El-Khoury, Pereira, Borgonha, Basile-Filho, Beaumier, Wang, Metges, Ajami, Young. (2000). "Twenty-four hour oral tracer studies with L-lysine at a low and intermediate lysine intake in healthy adults." *Am J Clin Nutr.* Jul;72(1):122-30. PMID: 10871570.

Evans, WJ. (2000). "Vitamin E, Vitamin C, and exercise." *Am J Clin Nutr.* Aug;72(2 Suppl):647S-52S. PMID: 10919971.

Field, Coakley, Must, Spadano, Laird, Dietz, Rimm, Colditz. (2001) "Impact of overweight on the risk of developing common chronic diseases during a 10-year period." *Arch Intern Med.* Jul 9;161(13):1581-6. PMID: 11434789.

Holl, Hartman, Veldhuis, Taylor, Thorner. (1991). "Thirty-second sampling of plasma growth hormone in man: correlation with sleep stages." *Journal Clin endocrinol Metab.* Apr;72(4):854-61. PMID: 2005213.

Kami. Hayakawa, Urata, Uchiyama, Shibui, Kim, Kudo, Owawa. (2000). "Melatonin treatment for circadian rhythm sleep disorders." *Psychiatry Clin Neurosci.* Jun;54(3):381-2. PMID: 11186123.

Lanzi, Luzi, Caumo, Andreotti, Manzoni, Malighetti, Sereni, Pontiroli. (1999). "Elevated insulin levels contribute to the reduced growth hormone (GH) response to GH-releasing hormone in obese subjects." *Metabolism,* Sept;48(9):1152-6. PMID: 10484056.

Koo, Huang, Camacho, Trainor, Blake, Sirotina-Meisher, Schleim, Wu, Cheng, Nargund, McKissick. (2001). "Immune enhancing effect of a growth hormone secretagogue." _J Immunol._ Mar 15;166(6):4195-201. PMID: 11238671.

Krzywkowski, Petersen, Ostrowski, Kristensen, Boza, Pedersen. (2001). "Effects of glutamine supplementation on exercise-induced changes in lymphocyte function." _Am J Physiol Cell Physiol._ Oct;281(4):C1259-65. PMID: 11546663.

Marharam, Bauman, Kalman, Skolnik, Perle. (1999). "Masters athletes: factors affecting performance." _Sports Med._ Oct;28(4):273-85. PMID: 10565553.

Marcell, Taaffe, Hawkins, Tarpenning, Pyka, Kohlmeier, Wiswell, Marcus. (1999). "Oral arginine does not stimulate basal or augment exercise-induced GH secretion in either young or old adults." _Journal of Gerontology. A Bio Sci Med Sci._ Aug 54(8):M395-9. PMID: 10496544.

Maxwell, Hoai-Ky, Christine, Lin, Bernstein, Cooke. (2001). "L-arginine enhances aerobic exercise capacity in association with augmented nitric oxide production." _Journal of Applied Physiology; Heart and Circulatory Physiology._ March;90(4):933-38.

Momany, Bowers, Reynolds, Chang, Hong, Newlander. (1981). "Design, synthesis, and biological activity of peptides which release growth hormone in vitro." _Endocrinology._ Jan;108(1):31-9. PMID: 6109621.

Rao, G. (2001). "Insulin resistance syndrome." Am Fam Physician. Mar 15;63(6):1159-63, 1165-6. PMID: 11277552.

Reaven, G. (2001). "Syndrome X." _1092-8464_ Aug;31(4):323-332. PMID: 11445062.

Robinson, Sloan, Arnold. (2001). "Use of niacin in the prevention and management of hyperlipidemia." _Prog Cardiovasc Nurs._ Winter;16(1):14-20. PMID: 11252872.

Ryan, Hurlbut, Lott, Ivey, Fleg, Hurley, Goldberg. (2001). "Insulin action after resistive training in insulin resistant older men and women." _J Am Geriatr Soc._ Mar;49(3):247-53. PMID: 11300234.

Rubin, Rita. (2001). "More people need cholesterol drugs." _USA Today._ May 16, 2001.

Sanders, Chaturvedi, Hordinski. (1999). "Melatonin: aeromedical, toxicopharmacological, and analytical." _J Anal Toxicol._ May-Jun;23(3):159-67. PMID: 10369324.

Suminski, Robertson, Goss, Arslamian, Kang, DaSilva, Utter, Metz. (1997) "Acute effect of amino acid ingestion and resistance exercise on plasma growth hormone concentration in young men." _Int Journal Sports Nutrition,_ March;7(1):48-60. PMID: 9063764.

Sytze, Smid, Niesink, Bolscher, Waasdorp, Dieguez, Casanueva, Koppeschaar. (2000). "Reduction of free fatty acids by acipimox enhances the growth hormone responses to GH-releasing peptide 2 in elderly men." *J Clin Endocrinol Metab.* Dec;85(12):4706-11. PMID: 11134132.

Tennessee News Service. (2001). "FDA urged to beef up statin warning." *The Tennessean.* Washington / Nation section. August 21, 2001.

Van Cauter, Copinschi. (2000). "Interrelationships between growth hormone and sleep." *Growth Horm IGF Res.* Apr;10 Suppl B:S57-62. PMID: 10984255.

Van Cauter, Leproult, Plat. (2000). "Age-related changes in slow wave and REM sleep and relationship with growth hormone and cortisol levels in healthy men." *JAMA.* Aug 16;284(7):861-8. PMID: 10938176.

Welbourne, TC. (1995). "Increased plasma bicarbonate and growth hormone after an oral glutamine load." *American Journal of Clinical Nutrition,* Vol.61,1058-1061. National Library of Science, PubMed abstract: 7733028.

Zello, Pencharz, Ball. (1993). "Dietary lysine requirement of young adult males determined by oxidation of L-[1-13C] phenylalanine." *Am J Physiol.* Apr;264(4 Pt1):E677-85. PMID: 8476044.

Chapter 4

Gastin, PB. (2001). "Energy system interaction and relative contribution during maximal exercise." *Sports Med 2001;*31(10):725-41. PMID: 115478894.

Gordon, Kraemer, Vos, Lynch, Knuttgen. (1994). "Effect of acid-base on growth hormone response to acute high-intensity cycle exercise." *J Appl Physiol.* Feb;76(2):821-9. PMID: 8175595.

Hennessey, Chromiak, DellaVentura, Reinert, Puhl, Kiel, Rosen, Vandenburgh, MacLean. (2001). "Growth hormone administration and exercise effects on muscle fiber type and diameter in moderately frail older people." *J AM Geriatr.* Jul:49(7):852-8. PMID: 11527474.

Jesper, Anderson, Schjerling, Saltin. (2000). Muscles, Genes and Athletic Performance." *Scientific American.* Sept(1)48-55.

Kadi, Eriksson, Holmner, Thornell. (1999). "Effects of anabolic steroids on the Muscle cells of strength-trained athletes." *Med Sci Sports Exerc.* Nov;31(11):1528-34. PMID: 10589853.

Lugar, Watschinger, Duester, Svoboda, Clodi. (1992). "Plasma growth hormone and prolactin responses to graded levels of acute exercise and to a lactate infusion. *Neuroendocrinology.* 56;112-117.

Roemmich, Rogol. (1997). "Exercise and growth hormone: does one affect the other?" *J Pediatr.* Jul;131(1 Pt 2):5S75-80. PMID: 9255234.

Vance. (1996.) "Nutrition, body composition, physical activity and growth hormone secretion." *J Pediatr Endocrinol Metab.* Jun;9 Suppl 3:299-301. PMID: 8887174.

VanHelder, Casey, Radomski. (1987). "Regulation of growth hormone during exercise by oxygen demand and availability." *Eur J Appl Physiol Occup Physiol.* 56(6):628-32. PMID: 2678214.

VanHelder, Goode, Radomski. (1984). "Effects of anaerobic and aerobic exercise Of equal duration and work expenditure on plasma growth hormone levels." *Eur J Appl Physiol Occup Physiol.* 52(3):255-7. PMID: 6539675.

Chapter 5

Bell, Syrotuik, Martin, Burnham, Quinney. (2000). "Effect of concurrent strength and endurance training on skeletal muscle properties and hormone concentrations in humans." *Eur J Appl Physiol.* Mar;81(5):418-27. PMID: 10751104.

Evans. (1992). "Exercise, nutrition, and aging." *J Nutr.* Nar;122(3Suppl)796-801. PMID: 1542050.

Hurel, Koppiker, Newkirk, Close, Miller, Mardell, Woos, Kendall-Taylor. (1999). "Relationship pf physical exercise and aging to growth hormone production." *Clin Endocrinol (Oxf).* Dec;51(6):687-91. PMID: 10619972.

Hurrell. (1997). "Factors associated with regular exercise." *Percept Mot Skills.* Jun;84(3Pt 1):871-4. PMID: 9172196.

Jakicic, Winters, Lang, Wing. (1999). "Effects of intermittent exercise and use of home exercise equipment adherence, weight loss, and fitness in overweight women: a random trial." *JAMA.* Oct 27;282(16):1554-60. PMID: 10546695.

Kanaley, Weltman, Pieper,Weltman, Hartman. (2001). "Cortisol and growth Hormone response to exercise at different times of day." *J Clin Endocrinol Metab.* Jun;86(6):2881-9. PMID: 11397904.

Li, Holm, Gulanick, Lanuza, Penckofer. (1999). "The relationship between physical activity and perimenopause." *Health Care Women Int.* Mar-Apr;20(2):163-78. PMID: 10409986.

Rodriguez-Arnao, Jabbar, Fulcher, Besswer, Ross. (1999). "Effects of growth hormone replacement on physical performance and body composition in GH deficient adults." *Clin Endocrinol (Oxf).* Jul;51(1):53-60. PMID: 10468965.

Sesso, Paffenbarger, Lee. (2000). "Physical activity and coronary disease in men: The Harvard Alumni Health Study." *Circulation.* Aug 29;102(9):975-80. PMID: 10961960.

McGuire, Levine, Williamson, Snell, Blomquist, Saltin, Mitchell. (2001). "A 30-year follow-up of the Dallas Bedrest and training Study: II. Effect of age on cardiovascular adaptation to exercise training. *Circulation.* Sept 18;104(12):1358-66. PMID 11560850.

Silverman, Mazzeo. (1996). "Hormonal responses to maximal and submaximal exercise in trained and untrained men of various ages. *J Gerontol A Biol Med Sci.* Jan;51(1):B30-7.

Widrick, Trappe, Costill, Fits. (1996.) "Force-velocity and force- Power properties of single fiber from elite master runners and sedentary med." *Am J Physiol.* Aug;271 (2Pt 1):C676-83.

Chapter 6

Bandy, Irion. (1994). "The effect of time on static stretch on the flexibility of the hamstring muscles." *Phys Ther.* Sept;74(9):845-50. PMID: 8066111.

Burgomaster KA, Hughes SC, Heigenhauser GJ, Bradwell SN, Gibala MJ., *(2005). Si x sessions of sprint interval training increases muscle oxidative potential and cycle endurance capacity in humans. 2005,* J Appl Physiol. 2005 Jun.

Dunton, Ross. (2001). *Masters Track and Field News.* Daily email edition, Wednesday, January 17, 2001.

Fowles, Sale, MacDougall. (2000). "Reduced strength after passive stretch of The human plantar flexors." *J Appl Physiol.* Sept;89(3):1179-88.

Hansen, Stevens, Coast. (2001). "Exercise duration and mood state: how much is enough to feel better?" *Health Psychol.* Jul;29(4):267-75. PMID: 11515738

Leach, RE. (2000). "Aging and Physical activity." *Orthopade.* Nov;29(11):936-40. PMID: 11149278.

Magnusson. (1998). "Passive properties of human skeletal muscle during stretch maneuvers." *Scand J Med Sci Sports.* Apr;8(2):65-77. PMID: 9564710.

Manchanda, Narang, Reddy, Sachdeva, Prabhakaran, Dharmanand, Rajani, Bijlani. (2000). *J Assoc Physicians India.* "Retardation of Coronary atherosclerosis with yoga lifestyle intervention." Jul;48:687-94. PMID: 11491594.

Roberts, Wilson. (1999). "Effect of stretching duration on active and passive range of motion in the lower extremity." *Br J Sports Med.* Aug;33(4):259-63. PMID: 10450481.

Tabrizi, McIntryre, Quesnel, Howard. (2000). "Limited dorsiflexion predisposes to injuries of the ankle in children." *J Bone Joint Surg Br.* Nov;82(8):1103-6. PMID: 11132266.

Sothern, Loftin, Udall, Suskind, Ewing, Tang, Blecker. (2000). "Safety, feasibility, and efficacy of a resistance training program in preadolescent obese children." *Am J Med Sci.* Jun;310(6):370-5. PMID: 10875292.

Wang, Whitney, Burdett, Janosky. (1993). "Lower extremity muscular flexibility in long distance runners." *J Orthop Sports Phys Ther.* Feb;17(2):102-7. PMID: 8467336.

Chapter 7

Antonio, Sanders, Ehler, Uelmen, Raether, Stout. (2000). "Effects of exercise training and amino-acid supplementation on body composition and physical performance in untrained women." *Nutrition.* Nov-Dec;16(11-12):1043-6. PMID: 11118822.

Gillespie, Grant. (2000). "Interventions for preventing and treating stress fractures and stress reactions of bone of the lower limbs in young adults." *Cochrane Database Syst Rev 2000.* (2):CD000450. PMID: 10796367.

Kanaley, Weatherup-Dentes, Jaynes, Hartman. (1999). "Obesity attenuates the growth hormone response to exercise." *J Clin Endocrinol Metab.* Sept;84(9):3156-61.

Kraemer, Keuning, Ratamess, Volek. (2001). "Resistance training combined with bench-step aerobics enhances women's health profile." *Med Sci Sports Exerc.* Feb;33(2):259-69. PMID: 11224816.

Marcinik, Potts, Schlabach, Will, Dawson, Hurley. (1991.) "Effects of strength training on lactate thresholds and endurance performance." *Med Sci Sports Exerc.* Jun;23(6):739-43. PMID: 1886483.

Medbo, Tabata. (1989). "Relative importance of aerobic and anaerobic energy Release during short-lasting exhausting bicycle exercise." *J Appl Physiol.* Nov;67(5):1881-6. PMID: 2600022.

Ronsen, Haug, Pedersen, Bahr. (2001). "Increased neuroendocrine response to a repeated bout of endurance exercise." Med Sci Sports Exerc. Apr;33(4):568-75. PMID: 11283432.

Sipila, Elorinne, Alen, Suominen, Kovanen. (1997). "Effects of strength and Endurance training on muscle fiber characteristics in elderly women. *Clin Physiol.* Sept;17(5):459-74. PMID: 9347195.

Sutton, Muir, Mockett, Fentem. (2001). "A case-control study to investigate the relation between low and moderate levels of physical activity and osteoarthritis of the knee using data collected as part of the Allied Dunbar National Fitness Survey." *Ann Rheum Dis.* Aug;60(8):756-64. PMID: 11454639.

Taylor, Bachman. (1999). "The effects of endurance training on muscle fiber types and enzyme activities." *Can J Appl Physiol.* Feb;24(1):41-53. PMID: 9916180.

Chapter 8

Cuneo, Salomon, Wiles, Sonksen. (1990). "Skeletal muscle performance in adults with growth hormone deficiency." *Horm Res.* 33 Suppl 4:66-60. PMID: 2245969.

Dintiman, Ward, Tellez. (1998). *Sports Speed. Second edition.* Champaign, Illinois: Human Kinetics.

Gaskill, Serfass. Bacharach, Kelly. (1999). "Responses to training in cross-country skiers." *Med Sci Sports Exerc.* Aug;31(8):1211-7. PMID: 10449026.

Kindermann, Schnabel, Schmitt, Biro, Cassens, Weber. (1982.) "Catecholamines, growth hormone, cortisol, insulin, and sex hormones in anaerobic and aerobic exercise. *Eur J Appl Occup Physiol.* 49(3):389-99. PMID: 6754371.

Medbo, Burgers. (1990). "Effect of training on the anaerobic capacity." *Med Sci Sports Exerc.* Aug;22(4):501-7. PMID: 2402211.

Mujika, Chatard, Busso, Geyssant, Barale, Lacoste. (1995). "Effects of training on performance in competitive swimming." *Can J Appl Physiol.* Dec;20(4):395-406. PMID: 8563672.

Nevill M, Holmyard, Hall, Allsop, Oosterhout, Burrin, Nevill A. (1996). "Growth hormone responses to treadmill sprinting in sprint- and endurance trained athletes." *Eur J Appl Occup Physiol.* 72(5-6):460-7. PMID: 8925817.

Sutton J, *(1976). "Growth hormone in exercise: comparison of physiological and pharmacological stimuli."* J Appl Physiol. 1976 Oct;41(4):523-7.

Track & Field News. (2001). Last Lap. "Super Bowl's Track Connection." March p. 49.

Vanhelder, Radomski, Goode, Casey. (1985). "Hormonal and metabolic response to three types of exercise of equal duration and external work output." *Eur J Appl Occup Physiol.* 54(4):337-42. PMID: 3905393.

Chapter 9

Barstow, Jones, Nguyen, Casaburi. (1996). "Influence of muscle fiber and pedal frequency on oxygen uptake and kinetics of Heavy exercise." *J Appl Physiol.* Oct;81(4):1642-50. PMID: 8904581.

Cook, Schultz, Omey, Wolfe, Brunt. (1993). "Development of lower leg strength and flexibility with the strength shoe. *Am J Sports Med.* May-Jun;21(3):445-8. PMID: 8346761.

Fuchs, Bauer, Snow. (2001). "Jumping improves hip and spine and lumbar bone mass in prepubescent children: a randomized controlled trial." *J Bone Miner Res.* Jan ;16(1):148-56. PMID: 11149479.

Kostka, T. (2000). "Physio-pathologic aspects of aging—possible influence of physical training on physical fitness." *Przegl Lek.* 57(9):474-6. PMID: 11199868.

Lemura, Von Duvillard, Mookerjee. (2000). "The effects of physical training on functional capacity in adults. Ages 46 to 90: a meta-analysis." *J Sports Med Phy Fitness.* Mar;40(1):1-10. PMID: 10822903.

Newton, Kraemer, Hakkinen. (1999). "Effects of ballistic training on preseason preparation of elite volleyball players." *Med Sci Sports Exerc.* Feb/31(2):323-30. PMID: 10063823.

Thompson, Glenn. (2001.) "Training Advice." *National Master News.* Feb.270: p.16.

Trappe, Costill, Thomas. (2000). "Effect of swim taper on whole muscle and single muscle fiber contractile properties." *Med Sci Sports Exerc.* Dec;32(12):48-56. PMID: 11224794.

Wheeler, A. (1986). "Isshinryu, one heart - one mind method." *National Paperback Books, Inc.* Knoxville, Tennessee.

Wilson, Murphy, Giorgi. (1996). "Weight and plyometric training; effects on eccentric and concern force production." *Can J Appl Physiol.* Aug;21(4):301-15. PMID: 8853471.

Winters, Snow. (2000). "Detraining reverses positive effects of exercise on the musculoskeletal system in premenopausal women." J Bone Miner Res. Dec;15(12):2495-503. PMID: 11127215.

Witzke, Snow. (2000). "Effects of plyometric jump training on bone mass in adolescent girls." *Med Sci Sports Exerc.* Jun;32(6):1051-7. PMID: 10862529.

Young, Skelton. (1994). "Applied physiology of strength and power in old age." Int J Sports Med. Apr;15(3):149-51. PMID: 8005728.

Chapter 10

American Academy of Pediatrics. (2001). "Strength training by Children and Adolescents (RE0048). 8/29/01. Internet: www.aap.org/policy/re0048.html

Borst, DeHoyos, Garzarella, Vincent, Pollock, Lowenthal. (2001). "Effects of resistance training on insulin-like growth factor-1 and IGF binding proteins." *Med Sci Sports Exerc.* Apr;33(4):648-653. PMID: 11283443.

Bemben DA, Fetters, Bemben MG, Nabavi, Koh. (2000). "Musculoskeletal responses to high- and low–intensity resistance training in early postmenopausal women." *Med Sci Sports Exerc.* Nov;32(11):1949-57. PMID: 11079527

Broeder, Quindry, Brittingham, Panton, Thomson, Appakon, Breuel, Byrd, Douglas, Earnest, Mitchell, Olson, Roy, Yarlaragadda. (2000). "The Andro Project: physiological and hormonal influences of androstenedione supplementation in men 35 to 65 years old participating in a high-intensity resistance training program." *Arch Intern Med.* Nov;13;160(20):3093-104. PMID: 11074738.

Brown, Vukovich, Sharp, Reifenrath, Parson, King. (1999). "Effect of oral DHEA on serum testosterone and adaptations to resistance training in young men." *J Appl Physiol.* Dec;87(6):2274-83. PMID: 10601178.

Cauder, Chilibeck, Webber, Sale. (1994). "Comparison of whole and split weight training routines in young women." *Can J Appli Physiol.* Jun;19(2):185-99. PMID: 8081322.

Dunstan, Daly, Owen, Jolley, De Courten, Shaw, Zimmet. (2002) "High-Intensity resistance Training improves glycemic control in older patients with type 2 diabetes." Diabetes Care, Oct;25(10):1729-36. PMID: 12351469

Escamilla, RF. (2001). "Knee biomechanics of the dynamic squat exercise." *Med Sci Sport Exerc.* Jan;33(1):127-41. PMID: 11194098.

Gibala. (2000). "Nutritional supplementation and resistance exercise: what is the evidence for enhanced skeletal muscle hypertrophy?" *Can J Appl Physiol.* Dec;25(6):524-35. PMID: 11098159.

Hurley, Roth. (2000). "Strength training in elderly: effects on risk factors for age related diseases." *Sports Med.* Oct;30(4):249-268. PMID: 11048773.

Izquierdo, Hakkinen, Ibanez, Anton, Larrion, Gorostiaga. (2001). Effects of strength training on muscle power and serum hormones in middle-aged and older men. *J Appl Physiol.* Abstract-A531-0. Jan. 29,2001.

Joyner. (2000). "Over-the-counter supplements and strength training." *Exerc Sport Sci Rev.* Jan;28(1):2-3. PMID: 11131684.

Kreider. (1999). "Dietary supplements and the promotion of muscle growth with resistance exercise." *Sports Med.* Feb;27(2):97-110. PMID: 10091274.

Jubrias, Esselman, Price, Cress, Conley. (2001). "Large energetic adaptations of elderly muscle to resistance and endurance training. *J Appl Physiol.* Abstract: 8:0057A. Feb. 27, 2001.

Koutedakis, Frischnecht, Murthy. (1997). "Knee flexion to extension peak torque ratios and low-back injuries in highly active individuals." *Int J Sports Med.* May;18(4):290-5. PMID: 9231847.

Mujika, Padilla, Ibanez, Izquierdo, Gorostiaga. (2000). "Creatine supplementation and sprint performance in soccer." *Med Sci Sports Exerc.* Feb;32(2):518-25. PMID: 10694141.

Panton, Rathmacher, Baier, Nissen. (2000). "Nutritional supplementation of the leucine metabolite beta-hydroxy-beta-methylbutyrate (hmb) during resistance training." *Nutrition.* Sep;16(9):734-9. PMID: 10978853.

Pu, Johnson, Forman, Hausdorf, Roubenoff, Foldvari, Feilding, Singh. (2001). "Randomized controlled trial of progressive resistance training to counteract the skeletal muscle myopathy of chronic heart failure." *J Appl Physiol.* Abstract: 8:0079A. Feb. 27, 2001.

Rennie, MJ. (2001). "Grandad, it ain't what you eat, it depends when you eat it – that's how muscles grow!" *J Physiol.* Aug 15;535(Pt 1):2. PMID: 11507153.

Ross, Dagnone, Jones, Smith, Paddags, Hudson, Janssen, (2000). "Reduction In obesity and related comorbid conditions after diet-induced weight loss or exercise-induced weight loss in Men. A randomized, controlled trial." *Ann Intern Med.* Jul 18;188(2):92-103. PMID: 10896648.

Schilling, Stone, Utter, Kearney, Johnson, Coglianese, Smith, O'Bryant, Fry, Starks, Stone. (2001). "Creatine supplementation and health variables: a retrospective study." *Med Sci Sports Exerc.* Feb;33(2):183-8. PMID: 11224803.

Sothern, Loftin, Udall, Suskind, Ewing, Tang, Blecker. (2000). "Safety, feasibility, and efficacy of a resistance training program in preadolescent obese children." *Am J Med Sci.* Jun;310(6):370-5. PMID: 10875292.

Stone, Sanborn, Smith, O'Bryant, Hoke, Utter, John, Boros, Hruby, Pierce, Stone, Garner. (1999). "Effects of in-season (5-weeks) creatine and pyruvate supplements on anaerobic performance and body composition in American football players." *Int J Sport Nutr.* Jun;9(2):146-65. PMID: 10362452.

Stromme, Hostmark. (2000). "Physical activity, overweight and obesity." *Tidsskr Nor Laegeforen.* Nov 30;120(29):3578-3582. PMID: 11188389.

Wilk, Voight, Keirns, Gambetta, Andrews, Dillman. (1993). "Stretch-shortening drills for the upper extremities: theory and clinical application." *J Orthop Sports Phys Ther.* May;17(5):225-39. PMID: 8343780.

Ahmaidi, Masse-Biron, Adam, Choquet, Freville, Libert. (1998). "Effects of interval training at ventilatory thresholds on clinical and cardiorespiratory responses in elderly humans." *Eur J Appl Physiol Occup Physiol.* Jul;78(2):170-6. PMID: 9694317.

Foster Higgins quote. (1992). "ASO's Feast of Services." *Best's Review,* August 1992. Cited in, "Movement to Self-Insurance Coverage." *Health Care* 1993. *Advisory Board,* August 1997. Washington, D.C.

Mathews, Howard. (1996). "Prescribing Exercise for your patient." *Maryland Medical Journal.* August. #45 (8): 632-7 National Library of Medicine, PMID: 8772277.

McGinnis, Foege. (1993). "Actual Causes of Death in the United States." *JAMA.* 1993. 270:2207-12.

Melillo, Houde, Williamson, Futrell. (2000). "Perceptions of nurse practioners regarding their role in physical activity and exercise prescription for older adults." *Clinical Excellence for Nurse Practitioners.* March 4, (2): 108-16. National Library of Medicine, PMID: 11075052.

O'Brien, S. (2000). "My heart couldn't take it": older women's beliefs about Exercise benefits and risks." *J Gerontol B Psychol Sci Soc Sci.* Sep;55(5):P283-94. PMID: 10985293.

O'Grady, Fletcher, Ortiz. (2000). Therapeutic and physical fitness exercise Prescription for older adults with joint disease: an evidence-based approach." *Rheumatoid Disease North American.* August: 26(3): 617-46. National Library of Medicine. PMID: 10989515.

Wideman, Weltman, Hartman, Veldhuis, Weltman. (2002). "Growth hormone Release during acute and chronic aerobic and resistance exercise: recent findings." Sports Med 2002;32(15):987-1004 pmid: 12457419

Conclusion

Desaphy, De Luca, Pierno, Imbrici, Camerino. (1998). "Partial recovery of skeletal muscle sodium channel properties in aged rats chronically treated with growth hormone or the GH secretagogue hexarelin." *J Pharmacol Exp Ther.* Aug;286(2):903-12. PMID: 9694949.

Godin, Shephard. (1990). "Use of attitude-behavior models in exercise promotion." *Sports Med.* Aug;10(2):103-21. PMID: 2204097.

Huddy, Herbert, Hymer, Johnson. (1995). "Facilitating changes in exercise behavior: effect of structured statements of intention on perceived barriers to action." *Psychol Rep.* Jun;73(3 Pt 1):867-76. PMID: 756803.

Lexell, J. (1999). "Effects of strength and endurance training on skeletal muscles in the elderly. New muscles for old!" *Lakartidningen.* Jan 20;96(3):207-9. PMID: 10068322.

Morley, Baumgarter, Roubenoff, Mayer, Nair. (2001). "Sarcopenia." *J Lab Clin Med.* Apr;137(4):231-43. PMID: 11283518.

Proctor, Sunning, Walro, Sieck, Lemon. (1995). " Oxidative capacity of human muscle fiber types: effects of age and training status." *J Appl Physiol.* Jun;78(6):2033-8. PMID: 7665396.

Stokes, Nevill, Hall, Lakomy. (2002). "The time course of the hman growth hormone response to a 6 s and a 30 s cycle ergometer sprint." J Sports Sci 2002 Jun;20(6):487-94.

Trappe, Williamson, Godard, Porter, Rowden, Costill. (2000). "Effect of resistance training on single muscle fiber contractile function in older men." *J Appl Physiol.* Jul;89(1):143-52. PMID: 10904046.

Turner, Wang, Westerfield. (1995). "Preventing release in weight control: a discussion of cognitive and behavioral strategies." Psychol Rep. Oct;77(2):651-66. PMID: 8559896.

Glossary

Aerobic Exercise - Exercise that allows your body to consistently replenish its need for oxygen during fitness training. It is performed at a low to moderate intensity for 20 to 30 minutes. Aerobic exercise is frequently called "cardio" and is used to build endurance and cardiovascular conditioning.

Amino Acids - The building blocks of proteins, which build and repair the body.

Anabolic - Growth oriented. The building-up cycle of the human body. Opposed to catabolic, the breaking-down of body tissue.

Anaerobic Exercise - The short, fast high-intensity type of exercise that uses oxygen faster than the body can replenish it.

Antioxidants - Compounds that lessen tissue oxidation and damage to the body. These small compounds assist in controlling potentially damaging free radical cells.

ATP - A high-energy molecule that provides energy to the body at the cellular level.

Atrophy - The loss and wasting of muscle due to inactivity.

Barbell - A long bar, approximately six feet in length that can accommodate weighted plates on each end. The Olympic barbell is the industry standard for heavy lifting.

Carbs / Carbohydrates – Nutrients supplying energy to the body expressed as "simple" (sugar), and "complex" (grains).

Catecholamines – Natural hormones produced by the body (adrenaline and norepinephrine). The body's release of "Catecholamines" during exercise is a growth hormone release benchmark.

Circuit Training - A series of exercises set in sequence. The exercises are performed one after the other, and typically target different muscle groups.

Concentric - The lifting phase when the muscle shortens or contracts. The "positive" movement of an exercise opposed to the "negative" eccentric lengthening phase.

Contraction – Movement of a muscle that results in shortening a muscle to push or pull resistance.

Cool down – The gradual slowing down of heart rate and body temperature that occurs between exercise and normal functioning of the body.

Cross training – The process of using several types of exercise in fitness training.

Dehydration – Losing too much body fluid during training. This can become dangerous if the body does not get replenished with adequate fluid during training. Dehydration will interfere with the release of growth hormone during exercise.

Dorsiflexion - Bending the foot upward during running to gain power from increased ankle action. Opposite of plantarflexion (foot down).

Drop Set – Sometimes called "Giant Set" is a series of three or more exercises performed in succession without rest between sets.

Dumbbell - A shortened version of a barbell, usually measuring about 12 inches in length, that allows an exercise to be performed one arm at a time.

Eccentric - The lowering phase when the muscle lengthens. The "negative" movement of an exercise.

Endorphins – A natural chemical released by the body during training. Endorphins are released by the pituitary gland and act on the nervous system to reduce sensitivity to pain.

Endurance – The ability to perform exercise for an extended period.

Exercise – Prescribed body movements intended to develop the body by working muscle groups.

Exhaustion Principle – A fundamental principle of Ready, Set, Go! Fitness, this is the point in exercise where you cannot physically perform another repetition.

EZ-curl bar - A specially configured barbell that has two sets of curves in the middle in order to reduce strain on the wrist joints.

Fat – An essential nutrient that is a source of energy for the body.

Fatigue - The point in exercise where the muscle begins to weaken.

Flexibility – The ability of muscle and connective tissue attached to joints to move in a full range of motion. Flexibility is increased through stretching.

Free Weights - Barbells and dumbbells.

Glucose – A "simple" sugar used by the body for energy.

Glutamine - An amino acid proven to be effective in increasing growth hormone naturally.

Glycogen – Substance formed by carbohydrates and stored in the body as an energy source.

Growth Hormone (GH) – A hormone produced by the pituitary gland responsible for promoting and regulating muscle and tissue growth, regulating carbohydrates and fat metabolism, and controlling other vital glands.

HDL Cholesterol - High-density lipoprotein. Also known as "good" cholesterol because it has scavenger abilities to remove fats in the blood. Exercise can increase HDL.

Hydration – Drinking fluids.

Hypertrophy - An increase in muscle size.

Hypoglycemia – low blood sugar.

Intensity - The amount of stress on the body while performing an exercise.

Isolation Principle - A fundamental principle of Ready, Set, Go! Fitness. This is the correct positioning of your body that allows one muscle group to be the primary target of an exercise.

Lactic Acid – The natural by-product produced by the body during anaerobic exercise. Lactic acid production in the muscles during exercise is the body's way of telling the muscles that there is not enough oxygen in the blood. The muscles begin producing pain sensations in a direct relationship to the amount of lactic acid produced. This is a GH-release benchmark.

Lateral - To the side.

LDL Cholesterol - Low-density lipoprotein. Considered "bad" cholesterol due to its negative impact on the cardiovascular system.

Metabolism - The chemical reactions that occur in the body. "Metabolic rate" is the rate at which the body utilizes energy. Exercise increases metabolic rate.

Muscle Pump - The pooling of blood in a muscle during exercise.

Muscle Tone - The condition of muscle that appears healthy and firm.

Nutrients - Nourishment for the body. Macronutrients are carbohydrates, protein, fat and water. Micronutrients are vitamins and minerals. "Essential nutrients" must be obtained from the diet.

Obesity - Over 30 percent body fat.

Peptides - Two or more amino acids linked together.

Periodization – A training method that varies training to prepare an athlete to achieve "peak" performance at the prescribed time.

Placebo - A fake treatment used to test research experiments.

Plateau – The halting or leveling off of gains in fitness and training.

Protein – The building block nutrients promoting positive growth and repair of body tissue. Proteins are composed of amino acids.

Recovery – Recovery has two meanings in fitness. (1) During training, "recovery" is the brief period between sets generally lasting one to two minutes. (2) Recovery is the period immediately following training typically lasting 30 minutes.

Repetition (Rep) - One complete movement of an exercise.

Resistance - The amount of weight or force used in an exercise.

Routine - The configuration of exercises - sets and reps - utilized in fitness training.

Set - A series of repetitions. Example: "2 sets of 10 repetitions."

Somatopause – A physical condition characterized by high insulin levels, low HGH, which leads to weight gain, increased body fat, obesity, high cholestrol, and heart disease. Frequently called *The middle-age spread.*

Somatostatin – A hormone that inhibits the release of growth hormone.

Static Stretching - Holding a stretching position without movement.

Strength training – Exercise to increase strength; weightlifting, resistance training.

Superset - Two exercises performed in succession with little or no rest between sets.

Symmetry - The way muscle groups appear to compliment one another, creating a proportional physique.

Synergistic - Parts working together and producing more together than individual parts would produce alone.

Technique – The form utilized in performing the biomechanics of an exercise.

Warm-up – slow and mild exercise that seeks to raise body temperature by one degree prior to fitness training.

Whey Protein - Protein and protein supplements that are made from milk.

Index

S

T

U

W

Best fitness book I've ever read. *This book is filled with detail and explanations that will be interesting and helpful to all levels of people. Whether you're looking to get in shape, lose weight, take your fitness routine to the next level, gain more strength, endurance or speed this book covers it all. The many illustrations make it easy to understand what the text is referring to. I really like the "total" approach suggested by this book. It addresses stretching, diet, strength training, speed and agility and much more. Well thought out and researched. A must have for anyone wanting to lead a healthier happier life regardless of your age or what shape you're in. - Stuart F. Scudder*

This is one of the greatest fitness books ever. *It tells you what really works and cuts through the BS. The author has trained many NFL players. It's very different from the typical exercise book that tells you to walk for 30 minutes a day. It points out walking is practically useless, as is loads of cardio work and long distance running if you want to get close to an elite level. – Jack Metal, Huntingdon Beach, CA*

"The information in it is unbelievably good...one of the best fitness books I've read...a classic. *I'm very happy that I found it. It's a great resource. - N. North*

"I've read your book twice now and I need to congratulate you on **one of the best books available** *for understanding what really happens when you train." - NASA Consultant, Jim Warren, President, Team America Health & Fitness*

"I've read a lot of books in my life, but your fitness book is one of only 10 or so that has had a very influential impact on my life. **I'm lucky I found it."** *- Mike Rabe*

This is an excellent fitness book. It is both well researched and well written. What makes this book so good is the fact that if you follow the program the author is outlining, then you will cover every aspect of fitness that is important, the author does not leave anything out. From weightlifting, to cardio, to stretching, to anaerobic interval style training, everything is present in this program. I have read many other books that make an argument that weightlifting is essential, but leave out how to integrate cardio work. Some books emphasize cardio, but leave out the short "sprint" style interval training that is so important to overall fitness. **This plan covers everything!** *- Anthony Yniguez, "Mr. Why" Catholic School principal Azusa, CA*

"I just wanted to tell you how much I am enjoying your book and your philosophy about exercise. It **makes so much sense** *and I can see using it to supplement and/or replace our current approach to working with many...if not all....clients." - Deborah Tregea M.Ed, Senior Exercise Physiologist* **University Fitness Center, Penn State Hershey Medical Center**

A few months ago, my doctor told me I had to make changes in my life. My cholesterol was high at 234, triglycerides were extremely high at 415, and as diabetic my A-1-C was 7.4. My doctor doubled my medication and informed me that my diabetes was affecting my kidneys. So I read Ready, Set, GO! Synergy Fitness and started the Sprint 8. After 4 months on your program, my cholesterol dropped to a normal rate of 141, triglycerides dropped to 276 (a 139 point drop and still dropping), and my A-1-C dropped to 6.4. I look forward to receiving even more amazing results when I return to the doctor after some more Sprint 8 workouts! Your program works!
- **Mike Campbell**

I read Phil Campbell's book a year ago and started the Sprint 8 program. Not only did this program help my fitness, it also improved my performance. The following masters track season, I received gold

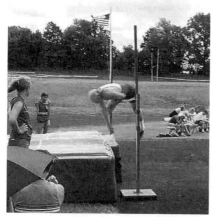

medals in the high jump and medaled in the 100 and 200 meter sprints during the Southeast Regional Masters Championships and the Tennessee Senior Olympic finals. This was the first time I had entered sprint competitions. My times dropped a solid .75 and 1.5 seconds in the sprinting events and I attribute much of this improvement to the Sprint 8 program.
- **Robert Southerlan**

Bob Southerlan, age 67

The information provided in "Ready, Set, Go" can be used to enhance any type of exercise program, from the simplest walk after work to the toughest gym routine. - **Charles Mills Editor, Vibrant Life**

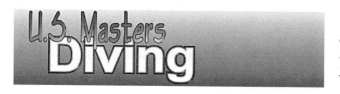

Ted Witte maintains an informative Web site for masters diving at
www.n2.net/diving

This is one of the **most logical approaches to fitness** that I've found. Not only is it full of step-by-step fitness exercises, but it goes into a great amount of detail about the nutritional synergy required to get the best results from a fitness plan. I have purchased a Vision Fitness Treadmill which incorporates the Sprint8 program and I am really thrilled with it. This is a great book! – Trader Tom,

I've been going to health clubs for 45 years, plus running for 22 years. While I'm in great shape, I had fallen in to an old routine. Phil's book gave me an effective new routine that gave me results right away - sprints, stretching, plyometrics, running, and weight training. Plus I have reduced training from 6 days a week to 5. Another day off with improved conditioning and flexibility. Very cool. **Documented programs for beginners to elites. Fully illustrated.** Of course it takes your time. (Less than I was spending before.) Of course it takes your commitment. Of course it requires your participation. Results or reasons. Take your pick. – Mike Hayden

This book lays out a lifelong fitness program and gets right to the point with excellent explanations and illustrations. Recommend to anyone looking for a simple yet complete fitness program. - Lee J. Ash (APO, AE USA)

I am **better now at 45 than I have ever been.** Sprint 8 has given me more energy and stamina to do all the things required of me. I especially appreciated hearing that stretching hurts him as much as it does me. I do it now and my aches and pains especially my back and hips are nearly nonexistent. I am a Master Herbalist, using natural medicine, I eat whole foods and follow Weston Price, and now I have Synergy Fitness, an exercise program that will take me into the second half of my life with strength and vigor. And I say Ready, Set, Go! A thousand and one thank yous! - Robyn Mulcahy

This **book lays out a lifelong fitness program** and gets right to the point with excellent explanations and illustrations. Recommend to anyone looking for a simple yet complete fitness program- Lee J, Ash